Transcending AIDS

University of Pennsylvania Press
Studies in Health, Illness, and Caregiving
Joan E. Lynaugh, General Editor

A complete listing of the volumes in this series appears at the back of this book

Transcending AIDS

Nurses and HIV Patients in New York City

Peggy McGarrahan

UNIVERSITY OF PENNSYLVANIA PRESS

Philadelphia

Printed in the United States of America

Library of Congress Cataloging-in-Publication Data
McGarrahan, Peggy.
Transcending AIDS: nurses and HIV patients in New York City / Peggy McGarrahan.
p. cm. — (Studies in health, illness, and caregiving)
Includes bibliographical references and index.
ISBN 0-8122-3203-8 (cloth: alk. paper). — ISBN 08122-1418-8 (pbk.: alk. paper)
1. AIDS (Disease)—Nursing—New York (N.Y.) I. Title. II. Series.
[DNLM: 1. Acquired Immunodeficiency Syndrome—nursing. 2. Ethics, Nursing. 3. Nursing Services—New York City. WD 308 M477547t
RC607.A26M386 1993
362.1'969792—dc20
DNLM/DLC
for Library of Congress 93-26279
CIP

Contents

Preface

This book grew out of research I began in the fall of 1989 and which I continued through the summer of 1991. I started with the simple notion that caring for HIV-infected patients posed challenges to caregivers, and I concentrated on nurses because "caring" is their job.

I am an anthropologist and not a nurse, and so I describe in this book experience that is not my own. I am the observer and the recorder of others' experience. I am also the observer and recorder of my own experience as the observer and recorder of others. This book, therefore, presents my own as well as others' understanding of the meaning of their experience.

That understanding took time. I had to learn a great deal that nurses take for granted. And I had to fit this new knowledge into my own conceptual framework, which then, of course, changed also. This meant that I often circled back to reflect on what I had been told early in the project, as my increasing understanding put what had been said then in a new light. The organization of this book mirrors this process. It can be read as my own journey, a journey from simple questions of what nurses do every day to profound ones about the meaning of what they do.

As I strove to understand what I was being told and what I observed, I was impressed with the similarities between nursing and the practice of anthropology. The most striking of these is the fact that intimate association with the "other" is a basis for knowledge in both professions. Anthropologists and nurses have to develop similar powers of empathy and cognition. It is through encounters with "others" that they both attain understanding. Thus I tried to make an unfamiliar set of behaviors and beliefs familiar by finding similarities within my own professional practice.

I did not read nursing theorists until after I completed my research and had written the first draft of this manuscript; I was anxious to keep my own view, as much as possible, independent of others who had tried before me to describe what goes on in nursing. I was pleased, then, when I did turn to nursing theory, to find my own understanding confirmed by writers with much greater claim to authority.

It was, however, in the encounter with what was dissimilar to my own experience that I found the greatest value. As I talked with nurses about caring for HIV-infected patients, I found that I had to think about many of my own assumptions and values. Not all of these were identical to those of the nurses I interviewed, and in having to examine theirs and my own, I discovered something more about myself and about others.

The nurses whose work I describe in this book were my teachers, and it was a pleasure to follow their lead. I can only hope that they found me an apt pupil.

Acknowledgments

The research on which this study is based would not have been possible without the generosity of the nurses I interviewed. They took time from demanding jobs and full lives to talk with me. I will always be in their debt. I can only hope that what they read here faithfully reflects what they conveyed to me.

The Greater New York Chapter of the Association of Nurses in AIDS Care (ANAC) welcomed me as an affiliate member when the chapter was organized in 1989. The help of the members of the chapter was critical to getting started and to completing this study. I wish I could fully express my appreciation of what they did for me.

Many others have helped me understand what it is I present here. Professor Shirley Lindenbaum, my dissertation adviser at the Graduate School of the City University of New York, encouraged and supported me from the first. Her keen insight, combined with good cheer, helped me bring order and structure to the project. Dr. Carol Germain of the University of Pennsylvania School of Nursing, my outside reader, was a meticulous commentator and critic. Her careful reading of the manuscript was invaluable, as was that of Dr. Ellen Baer, also of the University of Pennsylvania School of Nursing, who was the first to see and to help me see that what I was describing was the power and pleasure of nursing.

Partial financial support was provided by the Robert F. Wagner, Sr. Institute of Urban Public Policy through a dissertation fellowship research grant. I am grateful for their assistance and for their interest in my work.

To all who contributed to the genesis and progress of this project I extend my thanks and gratitude.

Chapter 1
Introduction

The Study

Human Immunodeficiency Virus (HIV) disease challenges the principles and practice upon which Western medicine has relied so successfully for a generation. It threatens many taken-for-granted assumptions and expectations. It cannot be cured, at a time when many scourges of former times have been virtually eliminated. It affects the young, at a time when most illness seems to be the province of the middle-aged and/or old.

For most of this century, the human life span has grown longer and longer, beyond even the biblical three score and ten. Now, with HIV disease, early death is again becoming commonplace. Before HIV disease, following the advent of antibiotics, infectious disease seemed inconsequential. Now, with HIV disease, infectious disease is making a comeback.

Most HIV-infected patients are young or in the prime of life, and yet they are almost sure to die. Many of them are engaged in sexual and/or drug cultures that are foreign to their caretakers. They may have no material or familial resources. They present many practical management problems.

The clinical parameters of the disease are not yet known, and success in treating the opportunistic infections that affect HIV-infected patients has paradoxically enabled the disease to develop new manifestations. The result is that yesterday's knowledge is often inadequate for today. Clinicians cannot offer treatment with certainty.

HIV disease has been called "an astonishing rebuke to a society and its health-care professions accustomed to the idea that the fight against disease is being progressively won" (Murray and Aumann 1987: 159). Yet for the nurses in this study, it also presents an opportunity to demonstrate the power of nursing as a healing art and the relevance of a social vision that combines humane caring with technical and scientific expertise.

The crisis of HIV disease affects all aspects of the health-care system, but its most direct impact is felt by nurses because they are charged with the personal, "hands-on" care of the sick. In carrying out this responsibility, nurses are continually making decisions—for their patients, for themselves, for the institutions they work for, and for their profession. Conflicts and contradictions occur because of differences between nurses and their patients, between institutions and the nurses they employ, between nurses and other health-care providers, and between and among nurses themselves. Professional training, experience, and personal preferences may or may not work together. Religion, gender, ethnicity, and class may or may not influence how nurses resolve the demands made of them. In addition, the media presentation of HIV infection as both a disease and a social phenomenon may or may not increase the difficulty of caring for these patients.

In order to deal with HIV disease, nurses must be able to tolerate ambiguity, uncertainty, and difference. They must be receptive to new ideas, new therapies, new kinds of patient-caregiver relationships. They must be open to their patients. Openness is possible when nurses view the patients they care for as people first and as social beings second. The "patient" is the "other," a human being in distress and in need of care. The care is given because the person is a human being and human beings—of whatever race, ethnicity, gender, or sexual preference—should be treated well. Thus, this concept of "patient" represents a moral commitment, a commitment encapsulated in these nurses' images of care. Using the category of "patient" enables the nurses in this study to overcome the fear, repugnance, avoidance, and hostility that normally arise in socially uncertain encounters (Perin 1988).

In meeting the challenge of HIV disease, the nurses in this study articulate and practice a philosophy of care that is based on a recognition of shared humanity between patient and caregiver. This philosophy enables these nurses to respond positively to patients who do not fit the American cultural ideal and to solve the dilemmas that arise from a new and devastating disease. It is a philosophy that reaches back to the beginnings of professional nursing but that also incorporates recent social developments, particularly the change in locus of decision making (Cassell 1991). It thus looks forward as well as back.

Models of medical decision making have until recently assumed that the physician, as the professional with the most advanced training, should have the final say (Reverby 1987; Melosh 1982; Starr 1982). For the nurses in this study, the patient should be the one to decide; the professional's role is to make sure the patient has all the information needed to make that decision (Allan and Hall 1988).

For the nurses in this study, nursing can be defined "as that service to the individual that helps him [*sic*] to attain or maintain a healthy state of mind or body; or, where a return to health is not possible, the relief of pain and discomfort" (Henderson 1939, quoted by Baer 1991). In a recent educational video, Virginia Henderson said: "As a nurse, I try to do for [patients] what they would do for themselves if they had the strength, the will, and the knowledge that a nurse has. And I try to do it in such a way that I don't make them dependent on me" (New York: NLN Video, 1990, quoted by Baer 1991).

Nursing in this context means acting with and for the patient in a manner that will enhance the patient's health. It is a comprehensive concept with few outer limits. How much is done for the patient will depend on the patient's condition, but at the core of this kind of nursing lies a connection with a patient, an individual human being.

Nursing can thus be distinguished from medicine, which is primarily the diagnosis and treatment of disease. Nurses "are involved with activities that contribute to diagnosing disease and they also activate many of the therapeutic mechanisms that treat diseases" (Baer 1991: 3), but their focus is on the effect of disease on the individual patient.

Nursing is also distinguishable from ancillary health care, such as that provided by physical therapists and social workers, by its overall responsibility.

> Nurses decide which care is needed by which patients, set up the plan of care, assign the appropriate level of personnel to give that care, and oversee it from beginning to end. This work takes knowledge, judgement, and a whole array of skills that are based as much in the social and behavioral sciences as they are in the biological and medical sciences. (Baer 1991: 3)

Nurses who embrace this conception of nursing must be competent in a number of areas so as to assess correctly what is happening to the patient and to act accordingly. They must be clinically up-to-date and responsive to psychological, social, and cultural influences on the patient's response to illness. Such nurses become interpreters to whom patients and other personnel turn. In fact, as Baer goes on to say, "nursing bridges the gap between people and science; nurses explain medicine to patients and patients to medical practitioners" (1991: 3). This kind of nursing is interactive and creative. It calls on all of a nurse's personal and professional resources. It is the kind of nursing that the nurses in this study practice.

For these nurses and for their patients, nursing becomes a joint endeavor in which they support each other. How this endeavor is undertaken and how it progresses, along with what it means for both nurse and patient, is the subject of this study.

I begin with the appearance of HIV disease in New York City. I then note the sequence of challenges this disease has presented to practitioners and institutions committed to the care of the sick. I consider how the philosophy of nursing these nurses profess enables them to turn toward rather than away from those afflicted. I describe what nurses gain from their involvement with their patients. Finally, I look at the cognitive and emotional skills that are required and reflect on what it is that HIV care makes possible, for nurses and for nursing.

What the nurses in this study gain from caring for HIV-infected patients is greater knowledge of other people, of disease, and of themselves. They gain personally and professionally from intimate association with their patients, supporting Merleau-Ponty's contention that "intellectual elaboration of our experience of the world is indissolubly linked to the elaboration of our interpersonal relations" (quoted in Malson 1972: 56). It is through the personal relationship with their patients that these nurses resolve many of the contradictions that affect nursing. In addition, nurses' contact with their patients expands their capacity for an integrated, nonlinear cognition that meshes rationality with emotion (Agan 1987, Sarter 1987). Their thinking about their patients combines scientific knowledge with knowledge about the patient's emotional, physical, and social state, so that the conclusions reached are not simply the result of a mechanistic matching of symptoms to solutions but also reflect the nurse's individual response to the "person" of each patient. Thus, in the act of caring, nurses create, however briefly, an encounter that permits the humanity of both patient and caregiver to flourish. It is in such encounters that the appeal of this kind of nursing lies.

It is my contention that the philosophy of nursing the nurses in this study espouse—similar to the philosophies of care that support other service professions—is a moral statement about human social relations. Caring for HIV-infected patients gives the nurses in this study an opportunity to turn this moral statement into reality. The opportunity exists because HIV disease is a particular kind of illness, because HIV disease presents a particular kind of patient, because the control hospitals and physicians normally exert is sometimes relaxed in HIV care, and because the attitudes of openness and accessibility these nurses exhibit find strong echoes in the current political discourse in New York City concerning the rights and entitlements of individuals.

In this study, I am primarily concerned with understanding the experience for nurses of caring for HIV-infected patients. It is an experience that requires nurses to face issues of human life that American society would like to forget: issues surrounding death and dying, sexuality and deviance, fear and abandonment. Through helping patients deal with these questions, the nurses in this study find that they too must confront these issues. What they do for their patients they do also for themselves. As Michael Jackson says of anthropological fieldwork, "the discoveries we make about others are valued only to the extent that we recognize them as reflections on ourselves" (1988: 205). In this process of mutual engagement with their patients, nurses become clearer to themselves. For the nurses in this study, the experience of nursing HIV-infected patients enriches their lives personally as well as professionally. Their patients become their mirrors, just as they reflect their patients' images back to them. In this "recurrent reflection" (Reik 1949), nurses become acquainted with themselves through acquaintance with their patients. As Reik said of psychoanalysis, "By taking it [the patient's experience] into ourselves, we learn something too of what is going on, or has gone on, in ourselves" (1948: 419).

As their patients experience change and development, these nurses also change. They and their patients become more reconciled to the human condition, to the existential fact that all who are born must die and that all must live with the knowledge that one day they will die. Through reconciliation, these nurses paradoxically affirm the value of living for each individual, even though each must die. This affirmation enables nurse and patient to relate to each other on a plane divorced from social definitions and ascriptions. This is transcendence.

Reconciliation and affirmation are not restricted to the nursing of HIV-infected patients. But HIV-infected patients, in their disease and in themselves, are more likely than other patients to trigger existential questioning. They compel their caregivers to think about human destiny and the social order.

Patients with other serious illnesses, of course, regularly die; they cannot all be saved. But the unremitting fatality rate of HIV-infected patients brings questions of mortality to the fore. In addition, the stigmatization of many HIV-infected patients, and the extreme poverty many endure, can be shocking to nurses who are, by and large, middle class and mainstream. Caring for so many who are so ill and so poor cannot help but bring to mind questions about the fairness and justice of the social order. The nurses in this study respond to these questions by transcending the social order and establishing a relationship with their patients based on the belief that all people have at least one thing in common—their membership in the human race.

As caregivers, nurses are participants as well as observers of the experience of illness. They stay with their patients; they are "there" for them. It is from their patients that nurses discover what being infected with HIV is like. For the nurses in this study, HIV-infected patients are the "other" whose experience can illuminate their own. Critical to that understanding is the time they spend with their patients. Time enables these nurses to know their patients well. Time also enables them to reflect on their own reactions to the patient and to HIV disease. In order to understand their patients, nurses must be attuned to their patients' points of view; they must integrate that point of view into their own understanding; and then they must serve as the translator for both the patient and the outside world. In so doing, a high degree of intellectual and emotional engagement is required. This engagement I call contemplative cognition. It is a kind of cognition that blends physical, mental, and emotional information. Nurses remain alert, attentive, and responsive as they use all their skills to understand patients and to devise appropriate plans for care. In this activity the individual nurse experiences wholeness, because she or he is able to combine domains that are usually separate. HIV care thus offers these nurses a special opportunity to experience integration of body, mind, and heart.

The particular kinds of empathy and cognition so important to nursing are not, of course, unique. Yet nursing does something more than use these skills. It institutionalizes them in the tradition of "hands-on" skills and in the discourse of "care." These are the practitioner's essential tools. It is through the exercise of these skills that nurses such as those in this study achieve their goal, which is to understand illness as it is experienced by the patient.

The viewpoint underlying this research is that a profession can constitute a way of "being in the world" and so can become, for its practitioners, a special universe. Committed professionals embody a particular set of principles and practices. For these nurses, who are committed professionals, their profession is not just "a technical task" but a "frame that defines a great part of their lives" (Geertz 1983: 155). This study seeks to illuminate the frame of the nurses in this group and to understand how the nurses create that frame. It is an attempt to "gain access to one another's vocational lives" (Geertz 1983: 160), and, in so doing, to render less puzzling the mystery of what other people do and why they do it.

Nursing is seen in this study as more than the sum of its tasks. It is "defined philosophically rather than sociologically, that is, defined by the ideal nature and purpose of the nurse-patient relation rather than by a specific set of behaviors" (Gadow 1980: 80). This study seeks to illuminate the nature and purpose of the nurse-patient relationship as exemplified in the care of HIV-infected patients. It is a relationship that "unifies and enhances the experience of the individuals involved rather than devaluing and alienating that experience" (Gadow 1980: 80).

For nursing as a profession, the debate over the care of HIV-infected patients has reactivated discussions about the spirit, the goals, and the techniques of nursing. Humane treatment of HIV-infected patients, like humane treatment of other conditions and of human beings in general, has to be fought for. Nursing thus has to be continually reconstituted and its meaning renewed. Crises such as HIV disease can be an opportunity for redefinition and recommitment. As Dr. Rieux, the hero of *The Plague,* says at the very end of the novel:

> Nonetheless, he knew that the tale he had to tell could not be one of a final victory. It could be only the record of what had had to be done, and what assuredly would have to be done again, in the never-ending fight against terror and its relentless onslaughts, despite their personal afflictions, by all who, while unable to be saints but refusing to bow down to pestilences, strive their utmost to be healers. (Camus 1948: 278)

My goal has been to present these nurses' experience as much as possible from their own points of view. I have sought to render what they do and the reasons they do it "from the inside" (Sanday 1983: 19). It is their story, told in their own words. And it is from the direct evidence of what they have said that the reader can evaluate how accurately I have interpreted them.

Above all, I have tried to present a full and fair description of what is involved in the care of people with HIV disease. I am particularly interested in how the understanding of what caring for HIV-infected patients means to the nurse is the result of a slow accretion of action, reflection, feeling, and thought. By focusing on the phenomenon itself, I have tried to avoid simplistic explanations of why these nurses have chosen to do this work and what they get out of it. Many domains operate at once in HIV care. It is this richness and complexity that I hope I have conveyed.

Methodology

This study draws on several kinds of information. First, and most important, it draws upon the personal experience of nurses caring for HIV-infected patients. This information I gathered in individual interviews with fifty nurses. I decided on the number fifty for two reasons: It was large enough to cover a wide variety of practice settings and patient populations, yet it was small enough that I could spend time getting to know each nurse as an individual.

The second source of information is my own experience as a volunteer in two New York City hospitals and as a member of a nurses' specialty association (Association of Nurses in AIDS Care [ANAC]). ANAC promotes the dissemination of knowledge about nursing care for HIV-infected patients and serves as a support group for nurses working in HIV care.

The information I gathered in interviews was later validated in a survey of the members of ANAC's Greater New York Chapter. In addition, I obtained confirmation for these results from informal conversations with a small group of nurses who met on a regular basis to discuss issues and concerns in their work. Finally, I draw on library materials as historical background to nursing in the United States in general and to nursing during similar outbreaks of disease in the past.

The interviews with nurses active in the care of HIV-infected patients were conducted between November 1989 and September 1991. The participants were volunteers, both to my study and to the care of HIV-infected patients. For eight of the fifty nurses, the care they gave to HIV-infected patients was a part of a general nursing position. The other forty-two chose to specialize in HIV care, although they were all in a position to seek out jobs that would not involve much contact with HIV-infected patients. This research was conducted at a time when nurses were in very short supply in New York City; these nurses could have changed jobs if they wished. Instead, they actively sought out positions caring for HIV-infected patients.

From my initial introductions to nurses doing HIV care I gained contact with others, many of whom introduced me to their friends and colleagues. Each nurse was asked a series of open-ended questions which led to far-reaching discussions of each individual's experience. Each nurse was then contacted nine to twelve months after the first interview for a shorter, follow-up appointment. Twenty-three of the fifty agreed to a second interview. Six of the nurses I interviewed read and commented on a draft of this manuscript.

The original and follow-up interviews varied in length from one hour to three. They took place in a variety of settings and at different times of day. Some nurses could only meet during working hours, others at lunchtime, some after work. We met in offices and coffee shops, homes and hospitals. The setting and the time naturally influenced the course of the interviews, particularly those conducted in work settings where interruptions and distractions could occur, but in each interview I encountered an individual who welcomed an opportunity to share and reflect on the experience of nursing HIV patients.

The interview format followed a regular pattern: I had the list of open-ended questions that I covered in each session [see Appendix A], but I was alert to ideas and topics that my interviewees were interested in discussing as well. I tape-recorded and then transcribed each interview and reviewed the transcripts carefully, coding for common themes and patterns. I used what I learned in the transcripts to add or expand questions in succeeding interviews (Patton 1990). I was thus continually refining the interview process during the research period. The responses of the nurses provided data which I incorporated into the survey I mailed to the members of the Greater New York Chapter of ANAC.

Using interviews as the primary source of data was particularly appropriate to the focus of this research and to the actual situation of the nurses in this study. The day-to-day experience of nurses at work is task-oriented, but the meaning of nursing is not revealed in an analysis or description of the tasks performed; the meaning lies instead in the integration of the task with the nurse's consciousness. This is not apparent in simple observation. It becomes clear through reflection, when the nurse examines her or his own reactions to what she or he is doing, away from the patient, the bedside, and the care setting. This is why interviews were a good vehicle for exploring the experience of HIV care for this group of nurses. They needed to reflect on and analyze their experience in order to articulate what HIV care means to them. Interviews gave them that opportunity.

Because the interviews took place over a long period of time, I was able to reflect on what I heard and to test my interpretations as the interviews proceeded. At the beginning, I simply sought to describe the experience of nursing HIV patients without prejudgment or expectations. I then isolated what I saw as particular to the experience and focused on how the nurses themselves understood this experience. Finally, I looked for the meanings that were not immediately apparent to the nurses themselves nor to me, but which were inherent in the experience.

In this process I followed the phenomenological method described by Spiegelberg, in which the goal is to focus first on the "things themselves" (1976: 656), leaving explanation for the final phase of interpretation. I tried to approximate a "first seeing" in all its complexity, before analysis and interpretation began. I paid particular attention to the processes through which the understanding of nursing HIV-infected patients was achieved, from that first encounter with an HIV-infected patient, to succeeding encounters that crystalized the experience in the nurses' consciousness.

My aim was not to dissect the experience into parts and to rank them, but rather to try and relate them to each other and to adjacent social and cultural phenomena. Through this approach I hoped to preserve and honor the multifariousness of the experience of nursing HIV-infected patients. I sought complexity rather than simplicity; I tried not to diminish the experience. And I used as my guide Spiegelberg's reminder that "the genuine will to know calls for a spirit of generosity rather than that of economy, for reverence rather than subjugation, for the lens rather than the hammer" (1976: 657). This method is a "determined effort to look at the phenomena [being studied] and to remain faithful to them while thinking about them" (Spiegelberg 1976: 700). It is attentive to the variety of modes in which phenomena appear and the greater or lesser adequacy with which we perceive them.

In this study, I am particularly concerned with the stages by which HIV disease established itself in these nurses' consciousness and in my own. What is in our consciousness does not appear all at once; it gradually takes form. The experience of caring for HIV-infected patients becomes increasingly complex to practitioners over time. And only with time does the meaning of the experience become apparent. I have tried to convey this development through the organization and presentation of the material in this book.

This study is thus a qualitative one. I use interpretive techniques that "seek to describe, decode, translate, and otherwise come to terms with the meaning, not the frequency, of certain phenomena in the social world" (Van Maanen 1983: 9). I am more concerned with ambiguity and particularity than with definitions and replication. I have, therefore, tried to avoid the constraints of "analytic labels, abstract hypotheses, and performulated research strategies" (Van Maanen 1983: 10).

Interviews are the core of this study but they are not the sole source of data. As I have said, I joined the Greater New York Chapter of the Association of Nurses in AIDS Care when it was in the process of formation in November 1989, and I continue to be an active member. ANAC is similar to many other nurses' groups formed around a specialty practice. There are associations of nurses in cancer care, intensive care, pediatrics, and so forth. These associations provide their members with contacts and up-to-date information, and they frequently serve as public advocates for the patients for whom their members care.

ANAC, as a national organization, seeks to serve as a clearinghouse for clinical knowledge about HIV disease. In addition, it operates as a kind of support group for nurses directly involved in patient care. It also speaks out publicly on questions relating to the care of HIV patients. For example, it has taken formal positions on the "duty of nurses to care" and on the testing of health workers for HIV infection. These positions were presented to the Centers for Disease Control (CDC) when guidelines and regulations were under consideration. The association, at its national level, also organizes an annual conference on nursing care for HIV-infected patients, while the New York chapter sponsors a local one for area nurses.

The Greater New York Chapter of ANAC meets once a month for a discussion of issues and concerns related to HIV disease, and it sponsors lectures on topics of interest to nurses taking care of HIV patients. The lectures usually focus on clinical topics, such as new drugs, the new CDC diagnosis criteria, or the identification and management of dementia in HIV-infected patients. The organization fosters social and professional contacts among nurses interested in improving the care of HIV-infected patients. During the course of this study, the association was helpful in providing me with ongoing contact with a group of nurses who report to each other about what is happening with the disease and with patients in the greater New York area. Thirty-three of the nurses I interviewed came from ANAC.

When the first round of interviews was finished, I sent out a questionnaire, incorporating what I had discovered in the interviews to all the names on the chapter's mailing list. Of the 170 nurses who received the questionnaire, fifty-six responded. These fifty-six were not among those I interviewed. Six questionnaires were returned undelivered. The completed questionnaires confirm the validity of the interviews. (The results of the survey are presented in Appendix B. A comparison of the survey and interview responses can be found in Appendix C.)

In addition, I met with another small group of nurses, numbering variously from two to five, on a more informal basis at regular intervals from April 1990 to September 1991. At these meetings, the nurses talked about what was happening on their units or in their clinics and how they were dealing with the challenges and difficulties of HIV care. This smaller group facilitated the expression of opinions and feelings that might have been unlikely in a more impersonal setting.

I also served as a volunteer at two New York City hospitals from April to December 1990. One hospital was part of New York City's municipal hospital system; the other was a not-for-profit hospital in Manhattan. At the municipal hospital, I was first a member of a team conducting a survey of HIV-infected patients. We administered a detailed questionnaire concerning each patient's personal and medical history with the aim of collecting enough data to develop a profile of the hospital's

HIV-infected clientele. As a member of the survey team, I saw patients in almost every unit of the hospital and I saw firsthand both the kinds of patients HIV disease brings to the hospital and the kinds of care they require. When the HIV survey ended, I joined a group working out of the Patient Relations' Office who surveyed hospital patients generally about the care they were receiving. This position enabled me to learn about patients' care in general, and, because I covered every unit, I was able to observe the interaction between nurses and patients within the hospital setting.

At the not-for-profit hospital, I was a member of the Department of Patient Relations staff assigned to welcome new patients, orient them to the hospital, and make sure they understood the Patient's Bill of Rights. Both of these tours of duty enabled me to observe the pace and organization of hospital nursing, the relations between patients and caregivers, and the special requirements of patients with HIV disease.

Finally, I spent several weeks in library research on the history of nursing in the United States. I gave special attention to nursing during times of outbreaks of infectious disease.

The Sample

The fifty nurses I interviewed for this study are not by any means representative of all or most working nurses in New York City. This is a small sample of experienced, highly educated, dedicated nurses who have chosen to do HIV care. Most of them are "experts" in Patricia Benner's (1984) sense of the word.

As can be seen from Table 1.1, the sample was 88 percent female and 86 percent white. None of the six male nurses was black or Hispanic. All were registered nurses, and more than half (56 percent) held baccalaureate degrees. Fourteen (28 percent) held advanced degrees. In addition, twelve (24 percent) were enrolled in degree programs at the time of their interviews.

All but two nurses were more than thirty years old, and most had many years of nursing experience. They were experienced practitioners who knew their profession and knew what they wanted from it. Before becoming involved in HIV care, they had worked in hospitals on general medical-surgical units, in high-tech intensive care, and in emergency care. One served as a midwife in high-risk maternity; others worked on oncology and psychiatric units. Two had recently returned from stints overseas, one in the Caribbean, the other in Cambodian refugee camps. Several served in home-care agencies. One was a nurse to a doctor in private practice. As a group, therefore, they represented a wide range of experience, yet each was drawn to caring

TABLE 1.1.

	No. in Sample	Percent
Gender		
Female	44	88
Male	6	12
Ethnicity		
White	43	86
Black	5	10
Hispanic	2	4
Age (years)		
20–30	2	4
30–40	26	52
40–50	19	38
50+	3	6
Degrees earned		
R.N.	50	100
B.A./B.S.	28	56
N.P.	5	10
M.A./M.P.H.	6	2
Ph.D.	3	6
Enrolled in degree programs		
B.S.N.	2	4
M.A.	6	12
N.P.	2	4
Ph.D.	2	4
Years of nursing experience		
1–5	6	12
5–10	3	6
10–20	26	52
20–30	12	24
30+	3	6
Current position		
Staff Nurse	22	44
Supervisor	12	24
Administrator	6	12
Research Nurse	6	12
Teacher	4	8
Current institution		
Hospital	35	70
voluntary	26	52
municipal	9	18
inpatient	16	32
outpatient	9	18
both	10	20

TABLE 1.1. *(continued)*

	No. in Sample	*Percent*
Home care		
not for profit	8	16
for profit	1	2
Residence	1	2
Research Organization	1	2
Education	4	8

for HIV-infected patients. At the time of their interviews, forty-two out of the fifty nurses in the sample spent one hundred percent of their time in the care of patients with HIV disease.

Most worked in a hospital setting: twenty-six in voluntary (not-for-profit) and nine in public (municipal) hospitals. This division was somewhat misleading, however, because ten of those working in voluntary hospitals gained their experience with HIV disease in the municipal system. As the voluntary hospitals began to organize HIV units and clinics, they recruited staff from the municipal hospitals.

Among those who worked in hospitals, eighteen were staff nurses, but six of the eighteen had additional responsibilities for case management, inservice education, patient counseling, and research. Eight were supervisors who coordinated care. Three were administrators, but one administrator was also an inservice educator, and another administrator had direct supervisory responsibilities. Six of those who worked in a hospital setting were research nurses for clinical trials of new drugs and treatments.

Of those who worked in a non-hospital setting, nine nurses worked in home care, three as staff nurses, two as administrators, and four as case managers and supervisors of field nurses. One was a staff nurse for a residential facility; another worked for a research organization, coordinating HIV/AIDS programs at city hospitals. Four taught nursing, three at the graduate level and one at the undergraduate.

Thirty-six of the nurses in the sample worked in Manhattan, seven in Brooklyn, two in Queens, and one in the Bronx. Two worked in Westchester, and two others in New Jersey and Long Island.

These individuals came to nursing from diverse directions. Nursing in the United States has traditionally been a female occupation, and the profession has frequently attracted ambitious young women from working or lower-middle class families for whom a professional R.N. license was a step up in status. Until recently, nursing was one of the few professions that welcomed women. The other career choices were elementary and secondary schoolteaching and social work.

For many of these nurses, then, the professions open to them when they were young were limited. They could be nurses, social workers, or teachers. They chose nursing. Some of them had been interested in nursing from an early age. They bandaged their dolls and treated them for ailments; they read Cherry Ames and biographies of famous nurses such as Florence Nightingale and Clara Barton. For most, nursing was also a route to a steady, professional job which promised financial security. For a few, it was a choice made without a great deal of thought. But all, at the time I spoke with them, felt it had been a good choice.

Most of the nurses received their initial training in hospital diploma schools and then went on to obtain a further degree. Others did not feel the need for another degree, and it is important to note that the hospital school diploma is sufficient for nursing licensure.

The sample is thus composed of highly educated, motivated nurses, many of whom hold advanced degrees. Almost all of them bring to the care of HIV-infected patients years of experience in other nursing specialties. They are mature, both professionally and personally.

That which truly sets them apart, however, is not their experience or their educational achievements. What they share, above all, is an unusual interest in HIV disease. Most of them sought out the positions they hold. This interest distinguishes them from many of their colleagues, who are either not interested in the care of HIV-infected patients or who actively avoid it.

They themselves note that they differ from many of their colleagues in their interest and concern for HIV-infected individuals. It is this special characteristic that makes what they have to say so important. They want to be successful in the care of HIV-infected patients, and they are in a position to consider—from the perspective of their own practice, past and present—what caring for HIV-infected patients means, how it compares to other kinds of nursing, and what it asks of nurses.

This study is not, therefore, a sociological analysis of "the HIV nurse." It is an interpretation of these particular nurses' experience. It focuses on the meaning of the experience of HIV patient care for these nurses, a meaning arrived at through the nurses' self-reflection and analysis. They, as well as I, were interested in finding out why they chose this work, what it offered when compared to caring for patients with other diseases, and what it might reveal about nursing's underlying mission.

There was no question I asked that they had not already asked themselves. This made them collaborators as well as contributors, especially as the significance of what they do became clearer to them and to me in the course of this study.

Chapter 2
HIV Disease and Its Impact on New York City's Health-Care System

The first reported cases of what would become known as HIV disease or AIDS appeared in the June 5, 1981, *Morbidity and Mortality Weekly Report* of the Centers for Disease Control of the U.S. Public Health Service. Five puzzling cases of pneumocystis carinii pneumonia, an infection caused by a protozoan parasite, had been treated in Los Angeles. The five cases were all young men and all were homosexual. As the *Weekly Report* noted, pneumocystis carinii pneumonia was a disease usually found in severely immunosuppressed patients. It was unusual to find it in five previously healthy individuals who did not have any apparent underlying immune deficiency.

At about the same time, physicians began diagnosing Kaposi's sarcoma in young, homosexual men. There were twenty cases in New York City and six in California. Eight of the twenty-six patients had died. It was unusual to find Kaposi's sarcoma in such young patients, and it was most unusual for the patients to die. Previously, Kaposi's sarcoma had developed in elderly men of Mediterranean origin and its progress was usually quite slow.

In response to the appearance of these ordinarily very rare diseases, the CDC in June 1981 began systematic surveillance for patients with these diseases. In July 1981, a task force was set up to characterize the syndrome (called Acquired Immune Deficiency or AID) that was responsible for the development of these diseases in young patients with no history of immunosuppression. The task force's goal was to determine the frequency of the syndrome's occurrence in the population and to find out who was at risk of becoming ill and why. The initial search was for laboratory-proven Kaposi's sarcoma and/or life-threatening opportunistic infections in previously healthy people between the ages of fifteen and sixty.

Meanwhile, investigators were finding this syndrome in other groups of the American population. During the fall of 1981, physicians in New York treated several cases of pneumocystis carinii pneumonia (commonly known as PCP) in heterosexual men and women who used intravenous drugs. The New York State Health Department reported a number of prison inmates with similar symptoms. The condition was also found in patients with hemophilia A and in patients who emigrated from Haiti.

Epidemiologists found it difficult to connect these different sets of patients in any way that would yield a clue to the syndrome's etiology. They had "no common medications, occupations, habits, or types of pets or any uniform antecedent history of personal or family illnesses with immunological implications" (Foege 1983: 9). What did seem to be common were behaviors that exposed the patients to blood and other bodily fluids. Multiple sex partners seemed relevant, as did anal intercourse. So did exposure to Factor VIII concentrates, a blood clotting protein. So did the use of needles.

Furthermore, what all the patients had in common was an immune defect that permitted opportunistic infections to take hold. These were infections that a healthy immune system could ordinarily successfully resist on its own or which, if they gained a toehold, could be routed by drugs. In patients with this new AID syndrome, however, these infections could spread and develop in unusual and alarming ways. The surprise doctors felt at the manifestations of this syndrome is evident in the following clinical comment about an early AIDS patient who died of a brain abscess due to *Salmonella enteriditis* and *Nocardia asteroides*, both common bacteria:

> This is an extraordinary case. Both organisms recovered from the brain abscess are handled by delayed immune mechanisms and [the patient's] delayed-type immunity had been vitiated by the AID syndrome. [The patient] manifested two of the most frequently observed infectious complications, pulmonary pneumocystosis and oral thrush, as well as an unusual superinfection due to a species of nocardia and a bacterial infection due to a group of organisms, the salmonellae, being reported with increasing frequency. The site of the salmonella infection is very unusual indeed. To our knowledge this is the first report in this population of a salmonella brain abscess and the first report in any patient population of a combined nocardial-salmonella brain abscess. (Louria 1983: 81)

In the absence of any identifiable agent, the CDC definition of this new disease in the 1980s relied on the presence of diseases indicative of defective cell-mediated immunity in patients with no known underlying cause for such a defect or any other reason for diminished resistance to that disease. Such diseases include tuberculosis (TB), oral candidiasis (a yeast), herpes zoster (shingles), and malignant neoplasms (tumors), such as Kaposi's sarcoma and various cancers of the lymph system. This syndrome was originally given the name Acquired Immune Deficiency Syndrome (AIDS), but with the identification of the Human Immunodeficiency Virus (HIV), it is now most commonly referred to as HIV disease or HIV. The appellation AIDS is reserved for patients with specific clinical conditions, either certain diseases or very low CD4/T-cell counts coupled with a positive test for HIV infection. (CD4/T-cells or T-lymphocytes enhance an immune response, limit an overly strong immune response, or attack and kill invading organisms and other infected cells.)

What HIV disease does, researchers believe, is remove the body's defenses against the onslaught of infectious agents. Thus, what in a healthy person would be a mild illness can become life-threatening in an HIV-infected patient. The viruses, bacteria, and parasites that cause local and limited infections in healthy individuals become disseminated in the HIV-infected patient and involve multiple organs.

In addition, few HIV-infected patients have single infections. They may start with a cytomegaloviral infection, which is manifested primarily by fever, weight loss, and liver function abnormalities. After weeks or months of such symptoms, a patient may go on to develop pneumonia or colitis. The pneumonia may be due to cytomegalovirus (CMV) alone but it is often mixed with pneumocystis carinii pneumonia. The colitis may also be mixed with herpes simplex, a virus that commonly causes blisters on the mouth or genital area, but which in HIV-infected patients can spread throughout the body. Mycobacterium avium-intracellulare (MAI), a bacterial infection usually associated with the last stages of HIV disease, has been found with CMV in the same intestinal tract, as has cryptosporidium, a protozoan which causes diarrhea (Armstrong 1983).

These infections are not new to medicine, and there are treatments available to counteract them, but their manifestations in HIV disease do not follow ordinary patterns. Both virulence and response to treatment are unpredictable, as can be seen in one of the most common infections in HIV-infected patients: candida (monilia), a yeast. Candida is commonly found in the mouth or esophagus of healthy people. In a patient whose immune system is intact, it poses no problem. In HIV-infected patients, however, the candida if untreated often multiplies out of control. It usually responds to orally administered, nonabsorbed anti-candida agents. But in some patients the infection persists until intravenous amphotericin B or oral ketoconazole is administered.

In others, the infection is never controlled and either persists during treatment or returns as soon as treatment stops. In still others, it seems to resolve itself spontaneously (Louria 1983: 74).

Unfortunately, the arsenal of drugs that has proven so effective against infectious disease in the last fifty years is relatively ineffective in the case of HIV disease itself. There are treatments for the opportunistic infections to which HIV-infected patients are vulnerable, but there are only three approved drugs that attempt to control HIV itself. One is azidothymidine (AZT), another is 2′,3′-dideoxyinosine (DDI). Both work in a similar way to prevent the replication of the HIV virus. Both have proved helpful in prolonging life, but each has serious side-effects as well. A third, DDC (2′, 3′-dideoxycytidine), has been approved for use in combination with AZT and DDI. None of these drugs is a cure.

Until 1984, a diagnosis of HIV disease depended on the number and kind of infections a patient evidenced. Then, in 1984, the identification and isolation of the presumptive causative agent, the HIV virus, led to blood tests for HIV infection. These tests do not reveal the virus itself; they reveal the presence of antibodies in the blood of individuals, antibodies first to viruses known to cause disease, and then to the HIV virus. Thus, these antibodies imply exposure to and infection with the virus itself. Several tests have to be performed before a diagnosis of HIV disease is reached.

> [T]he most widely used test, the enzyme-linked immunosorbent assay (ELISA) is used in conjunction with a confirmatory test, the Western blot, for HIV antibody; . . . A person is classified and notified as being HIV-infected after blood sample test results are positive in three tests—two successive ELISAs and one confirmatory Western blot (or another equally sensitive and confirmatory test). (Sloand et al. 1991: 2861)

There are gradations of HIV disease because HIV-infected individuals may or may not show symptoms of infection. For this reason there is a distinction made between those who are diagnosed but asymptomatic (HIV positive or HIV-infected), those who are HIV positive or HIV-infected and show only mild and transient symptoms, and those considered to be truly AIDS patients, whose condition meets CDC standards for a diagnosis of AIDS. Only the last group is considered to have full-blown AIDS, and this group is also now divided into those who are currently terminal and those who are not.

The CDC standards for an AIDS diagnosis are strict. A patient either must have one or more diseases known as "indicator" diseases *without* laboratory evidence of HIV infection, or must have tested positive for the HIV virus *and* have a disease associated with HIV, though not necessarily an "indicator" disease. Indicator diseases include candidiasis of the esophagus, trachea, bronchi, or lungs; extrapulmonary cryptococcosis; cryptosporidiosis with diarrhea lasting longer than one month; cytomegalovirus disease of an organ other than the liver, spleen, or lymph nodes; herpes simplex virus causing a mucocutaneous ulcer that persists longer than one month; bronchitis, pneumonitis, or esophagitis for any duration affecting a patient greater than one month of age; Kaposi's sarcoma in a patient less than sixty years of age; lymphoma of the brain (primary) affecting a patient less than sixty years of age; lymphoid interstitial pneumonia and/or pulmonary lymphoid hyperplasia affecting a child less than thirteen years of age; mycobacterium avium complex or M. kansasii disease at a site other than or in addition to lungs, skin, or cervical or hilar lymph nodes; pneumocystis carinii pneumonia; progressive multifocal leukoencephalopathy; toxoplasmosis of the brain affecting a patient greater than one month in age (source: *JAMA*, supplement 1S (September 4, 1987), 258:9, 1143–1145).

The diseases which can, *when combined with a positive test for the HIV virus,* be taken as a diagnosis of AIDS are as follows: bacterial infections, multiple or recurrent (any combination of; at least two within a two-year period), of the following types affecting a child less than thirteen years of age: septicemia, pneumonia, meningitis, bone or joint infection, or abscess of an internal organ or body cavity (excluding otitis media or superficial skin or mucosal abscesses), caused by *Haemophilus, Streptococcus* or other pyogenic bacteria; coccidioidomycosis, disseminated (at a site other than or in addition to lungs or cervical or hilar lymph nodes); HIV encephalopathy, also called HIV dementia, AIDS dementia, or subacute encephalitis due to HIV; histoplasmosis, disseminated (at a site other than or in addition to lungs or cervical or hilar lymph nodes); isosporiasis with diarrhea persisting longer than one month; Kaposi's sarcoma at any age; lymphoma of the brain (primary) at any age; other non-Hodgkin's lymphoma of B-cell or other unknown immunologic phenotype and the following histologic types: (1) small noncleaved lymphoma (either Burkitt or non-Burkitt type), and (2) immunoblastic sarcoma (equivalent to any of the following, although not necessarily all in combination: immunoblastic lymphoma, large-cell lymphoma, diffuse undifferentiated lymphoma, or high-grade lymphoma); any mycobacterial disease caused by mycobacteria other than M. tuberculosis, disseminated (at a site other than or in addition to lungs, skin, or cervical or hilar lymph nodes); extrapulmonary disease caused by M. tuberculosis (involving at least one site outside the lungs, regardless of whether there is a concurrent pulmonary involvement); salmonella (nontyphoid) septicemia, recurrent; HIV wasting syndrome (emaciation, "slim disease") (source: *JAMA*, supplement 1S [September 4, 1987], 258: 9, 1,145).

In November 1991, the CDC proposed new guidelines that would use as a diagnosis, in addition to the 1987 definition of AIDS described above, the number of T-helper cells, sometimes called T-cells or CD4 cells, found in a patient's blood. T-cells or CD4 cells are thymocyte-derived lymphocytes responsible for cell-mediated immunity. A low T-cell count means that the individual's ability to control infection is poor. A low count can be taken, therefore, as an indication of a defective immune system. Under this new definition, patients with T-cell counts under two hundred and a positive HIV test are considered to have AIDS, whether or not they manifest symptoms.

This change in definition has important repercussions for HIV-infected patients. It will expand the diagnosis of AIDS to many patients now considered only HIV positive or HIV infected because they have not had one of the opportunistic infections or diseases on the original CDC list. This change has its greatest effect on women, in whom the disease frequently manifests itself in gynecological infections and malignancies. Before the adoption of the T-cell or CD4 counts as criteria for AIDS, women with gynecological infections and malignancies and a positive HIV test—unless they also had a CDC-recognized opportunistic infection—did not qualify for a diagnosis of full-blown AIDS (Corea 1992).

The use of the T-cell count as a diagnostic criteria means that women suffering infections such as vaginal candidiasis, cervical cancer, and chronic pelvic inflammatory disease (PID)—which are not now recognized as AIDS indicators in the way that PCP and Kaposi's sarcoma are—will, when diagnosed with a T-cell count under two hundred and a positive HIV test, be considered to have full-blown AIDS. Some activists would like to see these gynecological conditions, without any reference at all to T-cell levels, considered sufficient for an AIDS diagnosis, but in the new regulations such infections of the reproductive organs in HIV-infected women must be accompanied by T-cell counts below two hundred to be considered AIDS (Corea 1992).

These new guidelines were to be implemented in April 1992, but objections were raised by public officials, health-care professionals, and AIDS activists that the new definition placed undue burdens on local and state public health departments, that it excluded conditions causing serious morbidity in HIV-infected women, that the emotional consequences of telling patients with low T-cell counts that they had AIDS had not been explored, that the variability in testing for T-cell counts had not been accounted for, and that the new definition jeopardized patients' confidentiality (AIDS ALERT 1992; Chang 1992). As a result of these objections, the CDC postponed the implementation of the guidelines and extended the public comment period, in addition to reviewing letters from health professionals and AIDS advocates.

In October 1992, the CDC announced a revision of the new criteria and proposed adding to the list of diseases which, along with a positive HIV test but without the requirement of T-cell counts below two hundred, would indicate AIDS. These additions were pulmonary tuberculosis, invasive cancer of the cervix, and recurrent bacterial pneumonia. The new additions are commonly seen in women and intravenous drugs users (IVDUs), two groups increasingly affected by the epidemic. These changes were implemented in January 1993.

The continuing debate about who is to be counted as a "true" AIDS patient reveals the slipperiness of the diagnosis. A disease entity should be well defined, but such is not the case for HIV disease. The move to make T-cell status the critical standard means that some people currently healthy are considered ill, while others already ill are not included in the same diagnostic group. The definition of health as the absence of disease no longer applies; the categories of HIV disease are distinctions of degree, not of kind.

The shift in CDC criteria is also a response to the change in the population groups infected with HIV disease. The disease seemed at first to be a disease of young gay men, and it was for a short time known as Gay-Related Immune Disorder, or GRID. The next group known to be infected were intravenous drug users. Some intravenous drug users infected with HIV were women, but the majority were men. Epidemiologists predicted that it would be through male IVDUs that the disease would spread to heterosexual women and children, and that has been the pattern. Partners of IVDUs are the largest growing number of HIV-infected patients in New York City.

Because New York City has the country's largest populations of gay men and IVDUs, it also has the largest number of AIDS cases in the nation. As of January 1993, 45,276 cases have been diagnosed in New York City. Of these, 37,037 (82 percent) are adult men; 7,194 (16 percent) are adult females. A total of 32,504 (73 percent) adult patients have died. In addition, there have been 1,045 (2 percent) cases of pediatric AIDS, of which 643 (6 percent) have died (source: NYC Department of Health, *AIDS Surveillance Update* [Fourth Quarter, 1992, issued January 1993]).

These numbers reflect the pre-1993 criteria for diagnosing AIDS. The new CDC guidelines have already altered the picture dramatically. According to Dr. Ilona Surich, the medical epidemiologist at the New York City Department of Health, the number of reported cases has

TABLE 2.1. Frequency of Diseases Diagnosed* in Adult Cases (diagnoses seen in at least 1 percent of cases).

Diagnosis	*Percent of Cumulative Cases*
1. Pneumocystis carinii pneumonia	55
2. Kaposi's sarcoma	12
3. Candida esophagitis	7
4. Cryptococcosis extrapulmonary	7
5. HIV Wasting Syndrome	7
6. Toxoplasmosis	6
7. Mycobacterium avium-intracellulare	4
8. HIV encephalopathy	4
9. M. Tuberculosis (extrapulmonary)	3
10. Cytomegalovirus disease	3
11. Lymphomas	2
12. Herpes Simplex virus	2
13. Cryptosporidiosis	2
14. Cytomegalovirus retinitis	2
15. Mycobacterium, other†	1

*Some cases have multiple diagnoses.
†Includes Mycobacterium species other than *M. avium* or *M. tuberculosis* or of unidentified species, disseminated or extrapulmonary.

Source: New York City Department of Health *AIDS Surveillance Update* (Fourth Quarter, 1992, issued January 1993).

jumped in the first quarter of 1993 by 100 percent (personal communication). Some of this increase is due to a one-time inclusion of all TB cases when the patient is HIV-positive, even those diagnosed in previous years. Even so, because T-cell counts are not required to be reported from medical laboratories, these numbers may tell only part of the story. In addition, there is a lag in reporting cases and some cases are lost in the system. Patients die of other diseases or trauma and are never diagnosed (Corea 1992).

The infections that AIDS patients in New York City have presented and which fit the pre-1993 CDC criteria are listed in Table 2.1.

These aggregate figures mask what are significant differences in the incidence of HIV disease in different areas of New York City. In the Bronx, the rate of infection per 100,000 ranges from 212 in Kingsbridge and Riverdale to 1,494 in Hunts Point and Mott Haven. In Manhattan, Chelsea and Clinton show a rate per 100,000 of 2,468 compared to 457 on the Upper East Side. The other boroughs show similar though less dramatic discrepancies. Some areas have three to four times the infection rates of others (New York City Department of Health, *AIDS Surveillance Update* [Fourth Quarter, 1992, issued January 1993]).

These differences in incidence rates follow racial, ethnic, sexual, and socio-economic neighborhood patterns. The Hunts Point and Mott Haven areas in the Bronx are very poor and almost completely black and Hispanic. Kingsbridge and Riverdale are middle class and predominantly white. Chelsea, along with Greenwich Village, which has an infection rate of 2,176 per 100,000, is where Manhattan's gay community lives. The Upper East Side is rich and white. Thus the incidence of the disease is not uniform across the city. Pockets of infection, where homosexuals, the poor, and minorities live, are interspersed with areas where relatively few AIDS cases are to be found.

Because HIV disease in New York City is at present a disease of marginalized groups, it has been difficult to rally people and institutions to the challenge the disease presents. Indeed, from the first there has been a tendency to believe that not only are these groups responsible for their illness but that they will be the only ones affected. As Kenneth Ludmerer notes:

> When medicine stands ineffective in the face of dread disease, the temptation to explain disease in cultural terms is pervasive and overwhelming. Society gains comfort and hope in feeling that outsiders or socially disapproved groups are in some way responsible for the outbreak of disease. If those groups can be placed beyond the pale of society—via stigmatization, isolation quarantine, or genocide—the epidemic might be brought under control. (1989: 9)

In New York City, as in San Francisco, the gay community has taken charge of the effort to make HIV disease an issue. Two organizations lead the effort to focus the public's attention on the needs of HIV-infected patients. The Gay Men's Health Crisis (GMHC), which was initially organized by politically astute activists, is the largest, best funded, best known, and most effective organization in the city dedicated to the care of HIV-infected patients. It supervises a raft of programs, mostly staffed by volunteers, which provide information on the disease, promote the cause of HIV care, and supply "persons with AIDS" (PWAs) with volunteer buddies who help them with chores and daily living. A more radical organization, ACT-UP (AIDS Coalition to Unleash Power), has organized political demonstrations on behalf of HIV-infected patients, pressuring governmental and medical bureaucrats to relax the rules on drug approvals, promoting needle exchange programs for addicts, and advocating the use of condoms.

Because the minority populations lack the community ties that enabled the gay community to organize its response to HIV disease, there are no comparable institutions in poor and minority neighborhoods.

There are efforts to set up education programs in minority areas, but most non-governmental organizations in these areas do not have the capacity to tap into funding nor to run effective campaigns for volunteers. The GMHC makes some effort to include minorities and women in its programs, but the majority of the patients they care for are young, gay, white men.

Both gay men and IVDUs pose special problems for care. New York City has always tolerated social behaviors that do not conform to mainstream patterns. As a result, New York City has a high number of single residents, many of them immigrants from other parts of the country and abroad: "Its percentage of unmarried men at the start of the decade was second only to San Francisco's, and the total number was far higher" (Killip 1989: 77). Intravenous drug users are also frequently on their own; the homeless crisis of the 1980s put many of them on the street.

Being sick without a family support system is difficult and expensive. Many of the services an ill person needs revolve around ordinary domestic requirements, such as cooking, shopping, cleaning, or paying the bills—services which family members ordinarily provide for the ill person. Without such family support, which many HIV-infected patients lack, the person who is ill becomes dependent on formal services, if there are any, provided by the state and/or charitable organizations (Vladeck 1989: 87).

The new wave of HIV-infected patients is equally in need of "homemaker" services. Women are currently the fastest growing segment of the AIDS population. They are also often the caretakers of families; when they become ill, those dependent on them suffer. Some have ill partners already; some have ill children. They cannot take care of others while they themselves are ill.

Unfortunately, the needs of HIV-infected patients—for ongoing care related to daily living in addition to medical treatment—run counter to the thrust of health-care provision in the United States. The American health-care system is organized around acute care. It expects that patients will be treated relatively quickly and released back into society, where they will convalesce on their own. The system is therefore unprepared to deal with an infection like HIV disease, which does not present clinically clear-cut health problems and which infects groups of citizens who need many and diverse services in order to live with their disease.

In addition, American public policy has always emphasized cash assistance over institutionalization: "The guiding principle has been to give people cash supplemented with specific services" (Vladeck 1989: 88). Patients are left largely to themselves to find and arrange for the services they need. Meanwhile the cash benefit part of the arrangement has always been low, because it is assumed that disabled people have friends and neighbors on whom they can rely for support. Since this is not true for many or most HIV-infected patients, this strategy falls far short of enabling people with HIV disease to meet their daily needs.

Furthermore, there has been a concerted effort, particularly in New York and California (the states hit hardest by HIV disease), to transfer as much as possible of the costs associated with the care of dependent populations to Medicaid. The reason for doing this is that 50 percent of Medicaid costs are paid by the federal government. Moving AIDS care, which is very expensive, to Medicaid, saves state governments a great deal of money. At one time it was estimated that the cost of care from diagnosis to death for the average HIV patient was more than $150,000; more recent estimates hover around $50,000 (Fox and Thomas 1990; Scitovsky 1986).

Even at the lower figure, the rising incidence of HIV disease means expenditures for HIV care must increase (Bartlett 1990). More patients mean the total cost will inevitably rise. In New York State, therefore, inventive programming has resulted in such creations as the AIDS health-related facility (AIDS HRF), which is "an attempt to provide a service that is essentially residential and supervisory in the guise of a Medicaid-reimbursable health facility" (Vladeck 1989: 90).

The consequences of this effort to define institutions as health facilities in order to garner Medicaid reimbursements are important. First, being a part of Medicaid necessitates a level of staffing, reporting, and oversight which in itself is a significant cost. Second, it means that the criteria for admission have to be clinical criteria, even when the circumstances that make admission necessary are nonmedical. Furthermore, as Vladeck points out:

> Ironically, it may also mean that residents of the facility get less than optimal medical care. As has been the case with nursing homes, policymakers require such facilities to provide a minimal level of health-related services in order to qualify for status as Medicaid-reimbursable health facilities; but they are then reluctant to pay for very extensive services, which would be irrationally expensive. In this case, the mediocre may well drive out the good: the provision of adequate medical supervision may in practice be more difficult in facilities with limited health services than in a purely residential setting into which targeted services can be brought on an as-needed basis. (1989: 90)

According to Vladeck, the effort to squeeze HIV services into the Medicaid box has distorted and delayed needed programs. In New York State, the primary responsibility for case management of persons with HIV disease has been assigned to hospitals designated as AIDS centers because the hospitals were already conduits for Medicaid funds. Whether hospitals were the best environment in which to establish AIDS programs, and whether the hospitals had the capacity to manage these programs, was not a concern (Levine 1990).

The state's reliance on Medicaid also has direct consequences for patients. In order to qualify for Medicaid, patients with HIV-related illnesses must either spend down their money to the poverty level or have advanced already to clinically defined, full-blown AIDS. Eligibility and, therefore, the criteria for eligibility, including the CDC guidelines for a diagnosis of AIDS, become part of the struggle for Medicaid reimbursement.

In New York City, a diagnosis of AIDS entitles a patient to special medical, housing, and nutritional allowances. The recent revision of the CDC criteria has doubled the number of patients considered to have AIDS. Whether this increase in the number of designated AIDS patients will produce additional services is not clear, given the current financial situation in New York City.

The gyrations state officials have performed in order to fit services for HIV-infected patients into existing health financing programs reflect the fact that Medicaid is the only mechanism currently available to pay for these costs. Medicare is supposed to provide health care for disabled workers who meet certain work history requirements, but few HIV-infected patients have received benefits because the Medicare application process for disabled workers is time consuming. It usually takes about twenty-nine months from first request to implementation. In twenty-nine months, of course, an HIV-infected patient may well be dead.

Further complicating an already complicated situation, HIV disease appeared at a time when the health-care system itself was shrinking. In New York State, health planners decided in the early 1980s that there would be declining demand for hospital stays and a corresponding increase in demand for ambulatory services. Between 1980 and 1985, therefore, eighteen hundred beds in New York City hospitals were eliminated (Killip 1989). As a result, hospitals in New York City show the highest average census figures of any metropolitan area in the country. Almost every bed is being used every day. Under the onslaught of drug abuse (particularly crack), AIDS, TB, and sexually transmitted diseases (STDs), census figures for city hospitals hover around 90 percent of capacity and a few report a census count over 100 percent. Such crowding results in poor patient care. As Killip comments:

> As anyone who is in the management of a large hospital (especially one with a busy emergency room) knows, when average census approaches 90 percent of capacity or above, the entire system is stressed. Flexibility to meet unexpected emergencies, such as equipment failure, personnel absences, or high volume, is limited, and patient care suffers. (1989: 76)

Municipal, city-run hospitals in New York City are particularly stressed because they provide medical care to the poor and minority populations of the city, exactly the groups most affected by the HIV virus. They are also the hospitals of last resort for HIV-infected patients who have exhausted their insurance benefits and/or personal savings. Municipal hospitals carry a disproportionate load. They have 8,288 beds, compared with 27,500 for voluntary hospitals, but in a census taken in 1989, 3.9 percent of voluntary hospital beds were filled with HIV patients, compared with 7.1 percent of municipal hospital beds (Killip 1989: 78).

In addition, the change in character of the HIV-infected patient from white, gay male to poor and minority IVDU and/or IVDU partner is a particular challenge to hospital management. When large numbers of substance abuse patients are admitted, "pushers begin strolling the halls. Wheeling and dealing goes on in the corridors and stairwells. Patients are 'shooting up,' and the atmosphere of a devoted health-care environment is easily subverted" (Killip 1989: 79). Before HIV disease, drug users were intermittent and infrequent clients of the health care system. They tended to come to the hospital for emergency treatment and then disappear. With the advent of HIV disease, however, they have become a large and growing percentage of all hospital admissions, bringing with them many management problems.

For nurses particularly, these patients can be frustrating. They do not conform to middle-class standards. They can be hard to reach, both literally and figuratively. IVDUs often lead disorganized lives, so compliance and follow-up may not be complete. They can be resistant to suggestion and persuasion. They may not have the educational background to understand explanations couched in scientific terms. This can make them suspicious of "the system." Thus, in general, teaching and counseling IVDUs about HIV disease and the kinds of behavior changes that prevent further infections are more difficult than with white, male, gay patients. One administrator of an AIDS unit told me that teaching her staff what to expect from and how to care for the IVDU patient was her top priority.

In addition, there is considerable distrust between minority communities and government in New York City. Some African-American groups have gone so far as to claim that HIV disease is a form of genocide through the introduction of disease into a vulnerable population (Dumpson et al. 1989). This complicates care in many ways. Patients come to the hospital because there is nowhere else to go, but they may not be candid about their histories and may not be receptive to the recommendations of the staff.

From a number of directions, therefore, hospitals are under increased and unremitting stress, as are the personnel who staff them. HIV disease is not the only source of this stress, but HIV disease in New York City, both because of its nature and because of the patients affected, has made visible the fragmentation and disarray of the health care system. Simply stated, health care for the poor is not the same as health care for the rich. Neither is it the same for groups outside the boundaries of mainstream culture. The effort to provide care for the poor and marginalized, limited as it is, puts enormous strain on an already overburdened system.

Health care never operates in a vacuum; its provision depends on the larger social environment where political decisions are made. The care of HIV-infected patients is affected by social and political currents within the body politic and is subject to the ongoing debates and divisions within the health-care system itself. These debates center on access to care. Unless an individual is rich enough to pay for care without recourse to an insurance plan or is insured under a health plan sponsored by an employer, the only care available to an HIV-infected patient is that provided by public institutions. HIV-infected patients in New York State become eligible for Medicaid, if they are not already enrolled before becoming infected, when they are deemed disabled.

In New York City, the system of municipal hospitals, publicly funded, takes care of all in need; no one unable to produce a cash deposit or an insurance or Medicaid card is turned away. But because the demand for care is always greater than the supply, the wait for care can be long, whether in the emergency room, the clinic, or the ward. And because these hospitals are under constant pressure to cut costs, the level of care may be minimal.

In the 1980s, just when HIV disease began to make its presence felt, cost-containment measures, specifically DRGs (Diagnosis Related Groups), prompted severe cost cutting. Hospitals moved briskly into ambulatory care, cut the number of days patients could stay, and generally increased the pressure on personnel to do more in less time.

New York City hospitals, municipal and voluntary (non-profit), have the lowest financial operating margins in the country (Killip 1989) and therefore have felt the greatest incentive to find ways to control costs.

The combination of cost-cutting and the emergence of HIV disease plunged New York City hospitals into a difficult time in the 1980s. Demands for care swiftly outpaced resources. The situation in many hospitals became chaotic. By 1987, fifty-two percent of all admissions to these hospitals were unscheduled; patients simply appeared, without records, without workups. Sixty-six percent of admissions to municipal hospitals and 46 percent of admissions to voluntary hospitals came through the emergency room. Such a situation made anticipation difficult and planning an exercise in hope, if not an exercise in futility. In 1987, the Bigel Institute for Health Policy issued a report on health care in New York City that documented the conditions under which the system was struggling. The situation was described as "medical gridlock" (Killip 1989).

Hospital personnel were the first to feel the contraction of funds in the health-care system—because low operating margins mean "a continuous scrutiny of personnel costs, the largest item in any hospital budget" (Killip 1990: 76). Layoffs meant that there were fewer people to perform the tasks needed. Patients found that appointments had to be scheduled weeks, sometimes months, ahead. Higher patient-caregiver ratios for inpatient units were established, and with same-day admission for many procedures and shorter stays in hospitals overall, nursing staffs particularly found that there was less time available to do all that had to be done. One nurse in this study described the New York City health-care system as:

> a deprived system because resources are always dwindling. We have to be more and more resourceful about getting the things we need. It's not supplies; we have enough gloves, etc. It's that we have no space, no privacy, no place to interview patients. And some of the niceties, some of the things which would make being sick and in the hospital more bearable, are missing. Here [in a municipal hospital] we don't have enough sheets and there aren't enough pillows. The pillows walk out the door. We use paper towels now because the towels were all stolen. The food is dreadful. I feel badly for our patients who have to spend, sometimes, months in the hospital.

The deterioration of the health-care system has placed a particular strain on nurses. Nurses are the links between the individual patient and the health-care system. The system does not provide them with all the resources they need, yet they have to work within it. They have a great deal to do and not enough time to do it. There is continual pressure to complete tasks quickly and to move on to the next. The temptation to treat patients as tasks to be finished rather than as people to be cared for is strong. Many of the nurses in this study could not find time for a second interview with me because their workloads had increased so substantially since I first spoke with them.

Providing care within a health-care system beset by social and financial challenge is not easy. HIV disease has brought into this system patients who need an extraordinary concentration of care, yet who do not represent what is culturally valued in American society. They challenge America's faith in medicine as well as conventional notions of social worth (Jonsen 1990; Schwarz 1989).

HIV disease may be a catalyst for further fragmentation of the health-care system. It disturbs the way care has been paid for, it evades the arsenal that medicine uses against it, and it brings into the hospitals and clinics groups of patients who have not, until now, been visible in the system. HIV disease upsets usual practices, cognitive habits, and affective inclinations by asking who is worthy of care, what kind of care should be provided, who should do it, and who should pay for it.

Yet, paradoxically, it is because HIV disease disturbs the usual way of doing things that the nurses in this study find the care of HIV-infected patients so satisfying. Disturbance in this case brings freedom, which for these nurses means the opportunity to practice nursing according to their own standards, not the institution's. The women and men in this study, therefore, have not succumbed to the personal and institutional malaise that dominates the response to HIV disease in so many situations. That they have not is a tribute to their training and their tenacity. It is also true that their perseverance brings them great intellectual and emotional rewards.

Chapter 3
First Encounters with the Disease: Choosing to Care for HIV-Infected Patients

By now, in 1993, HIV disease is well known. It has had a name for almost a decade; its causative agent has been identified to the satisfaction of most, if not all (Heimhoff and Sommer 1991: Cantwell 1983) practitioners; and each year adds something to what has already been established.

At the beginning, however, there was simply the sense on the part of many nurses that something unusual was going on. Patients came into the hospital with pneumonia and died when they shouldn't have. They wasted away. They developed unusual cancers. They had fevers that went right off the charts. And they were young. At first, there weren't enough of them to attract the attention of epidemiologists; they were scattered in different hospitals, and until 1981, when the CDC started its surveillance, no one was collecting data on a systematic basis. The New York City *AIDS Surveillance Reports* note only forty-six cases of AIDS before 1981.

But these patients who puzzled their caregivers stayed in nurses' consciousnesses. They were the patients nurses wondered about later, when HIV disease was identified. To many of their nurses, it seemed clear that these patients must have been infected with the HIV virus. Bette V., a nurse who went on to become the head of an AIDS unit and then a director of nursing in a voluntary hospital, recalled the era of the earliest HIV patients:

> In 1980, when the first AIDS patients arrived, no one knew what it was. It was labeled "Fever of Unknown Origin." Patients were almost entirely young men in their mid- to late-twenties who would come in

> unable to breathe, and they would get oxygen masks, and we would increase the oxygen, and then they would be dead, like in two weeks. . . . There weren't many at the beginning, and they were really all young, healthy people who suddenly couldn't walk up a flight of stairs and became rapidly ill. They ended up on respirators in the intensive care unit, and then they died, because we really didn't realize what was going on. The bacteria, well, now they think it's a fungus, get into the lungs and make them fibrous so the oxygen can't get through; so no matter what we did for them, they couldn't get any air into their bodies. It was really something. They had terrible fevers which we couldn't control, because they weren't from anything we could treat with antibiotics. So they would get every drug, and still nothing would work. It was pretty horrifying.

For Alice D., at the time in private practice with a physician in lower Manhattan, the appearance of HIV disease followed a decade of seeing an increase in venereal disease. Her patients were almost all gay white men who lived in the Greenwich Village–Chelsea area, among whom sexually transmitted diseases were commonplace in the 1970s. Then, quite suddenly, many of her patients began to present puzzling symptoms, different from the usual symptoms of venereal disease. She said of that time:

> There was a lot of coming out of the closet, and there was a lot of celebration of the change in lifestyle, of people who had heretofore felt very much repressed and ashamed. And as a result of that, we saw a lot of venereal disease, STDs as they are now called. That was throughout the seventies, and then in late 1980, we saw symptoms of a disease that we didn't know how to diagnose; we didn't know what was going on. I think our first patient had, in retrospect, PCP, and of course people get pneumonia all the time. That's nothing uncommon. But this was a particular type of pneumonia that you just don't see in people who are not immunocompromised for some other reason. I think our next patient had KS, and again we looked it up in the medical books, and until recently that had been a disease of mainly elderly men of Mediterranean origin. Young people weren't supposed to get it. Then many of our patients whom we had seen for years on a very regular basis, treating their gonorrhea and their hepatitis and their ghiardia—and other diseases which I had not heard of before I came to work in this practice—all of a sudden they were coming in with unusual symptoms. They were losing weight, and their blood counts were falling. In a fairly short time, we learned

> to run T-cell counts, and we found that their T-cell counts were low. Then word started filtering through this [gay] community that there was some strange new disease going on.

These patients with mysterious ailments, with gastro-intestinal disorders and respiratory difficulties for which nothing worked, linger in their nurses' memories. They were the vanguard of the present epidemic. But it was not apparent at the beginning how serious the disease might be or how many might be involved. These were simply individuals whose symptoms did not respond to treatment. There was no suggestion that treatment might not be available. Marcia B., who was working at the time in a Manhattan emergency room in the East Village, described what she considers her first HIV-infected patient:

> One weekday evening I was in the ER and he came in with diarrhea; he was a German immigrant, a frightened little rabbit with incredible blue eyes, and since we didn't know what was causing the diarrhea, we thought it might be Crohn's disease. We put him on hepatitis precautions. He was in for a couple of weeks, and I think the staff really mothered him. His English wasn't good, he didn't communicate that well and he looked frightened all the time. This huge black man who was his pimp came in and we became very protective of ———. He was worked up and he was discharged with some steroid for Crohn's disease, and he was out for about two months. Then he came back in, and he was on the floor for about three months, just getting sicker and sicker. Every specialist down there came in to see him. Finally, we transferred him to the ICU; he was just deteriorating awfully. No one could figure out what was wrong with him; he was in the medical ICU for three weeks before he died, and then we got the autopsy. It showed his whole body was invaded with herpes. The colon was perfect.

The frustration for the nurse in trying to deal with a disease that resisted treatment was often matched by the frustration of the patient for whom no treatment worked. Roberta S., who was just at the beginning of her nursing career in 1981, remembers one case:

> We had this patient, he was black, and he was a drug addict, and that was something I don't think he knew we knew. I just remember him being so frustrated himself at no one being able to figure out what was wrong with him. They ran every test imaginable, and couldn't find an answer. His temperature kept going way up, but we couldn't find anything. He didn't look like a person who was infected. A lot of

people, when they're infected, they're kind of lethargic and lying in bed, and they know where they hurt. The blood count's real high, and we give them an antibiotic, and then they get well. That's an infection. But this guy had all these high fevers, and it wasn't showing the picture of infection. I don't remember what his blood counts were, but I do remember how sick he was; he couldn't get well, and he was so frustrated. Every day I would come in and hope that yesterday's test had found something, and I remember getting frustrated myself, and feeling his frustration, until the day I came in and that was it. He had died. He died trying to find out what was wrong with him. They couldn't find what in the world was the matter with him. He just kept getting skinnier and skinnier and skinnier and he never got well. We'd given him everything in the world. He couldn't hold any food down either, and he had all that diarrhea.

These patients with conditions that fit no known disease entity puzzled health professionals, and the search for an explanation quickly took hold. As Alice D. said of her experience:

> All of a sudden, the doctor I was working with started hearing from other doctors that they too were seeing patients with these strange symptoms, and so we all started putting two and two together and came to the conclusion that this was a new disease and the only thing our patients had in common was that they were gay men.

The recognition that this was a new disease is forever associated for Alice D. with the weekend of July 4, 1981:

> I remember the date because that weekend I happened to be visiting friends in the country, and I was telling them about this strange new cancer that we were seeing in gay men, and they started rolling their eyes around and saying "you're making this up," and then it came out in the *New York Times*. And it was the first time it hit the mass media that something was going on.

But having a name and the recognition of a new disease, when treatment did little to help, was a dubious advance. Now patients had an identifiable condition, but the reality was that they continued to suffer without much hope of relief. As Alice D. went on to say:

> After that [the announcement in the newspapers], we started getting a lot of hysterical patients who were scared to death, and there was a lot of denial. They couldn't imagine how this could possibly be

happening to them and to their community. Many people did not change their lifestyle, and no one could figure out why some came down with it [HIV disease] and some did not, although their lifestyles seemed to be the same.

At that time, the HIV virus had not been isolated, so the search for an explanation led Alice D. and the physician she practiced with to do an epidemiological study, trying to establish connections that would clarify the cause of this new disease. She said:

It was exactly like being detectives. We were looking for clues everywhere. We decided that it must be something sexually transmitted, so we did a study in which we plotted the sexual activities, the frequency and the number of partners of gay men with their T-cell counts, and of course there was an inverse correlation between their T-cell count and the number of partners. We got good information; we really felt that the participants in our study were very straightforward.

The first patients identified as HIV-infected made strong impressions on these nurses. For Frances L., who was no older than most of these patients, her first HIV-infected patient

was a young guy who was a dancer. He had Kaposi's sarcoma, where they get the big purple patches. I remember him so well; he had them in his rectum, it was just terrible, because I remember he had these beautiful long legs, and I just remember him lying in bed, in pain.

The numbers of these patients grew inexorably, from 143 reported in 1981 to a peak of 6000 plus in both 1988 and 1989 (New York City Department of Health, *AIDS Surveillance Report* [June 1990: 4]). It was no longer an isolated patient here or there who baffled medical diagnosis. It became, over the course of just four years, when reported cases moved from low three-digit to high four-digit numbers, a group of patients whose medical and social characteristics required an extraordinary response.

HIV disease, like most serious diseases, is an assault on the patient's body as well as on the patient's sense of self. But because HIV disease attacks in a multitude of ways, and because it is exceptionally virulent, its effects can be overwhelming both for patient and nurse. As Carol H., a nurse with more than twenty-five years of experience, said:

> I think the thing that I found about HIV disease, more than cancer or anything else, is that it's the nastiest disease. It seems to affect everything, and it's so degrading to have it. You're not allowed any dignity, and [for] certain people, like gay people, who are very tied up with their appearance, it can be awful because many of them have KS, but even if they don't, it's not a pretty disease.

It is a disease that frequently leaves the patient with little dignity at the end. They become totally dependent on their caregivers for the basic routines of life. This is one aspect of the disease that evokes strong feelings of pity and horror and anger. Meeting that first patient in the end stages can be a searing experience. Lena F. met her first HIV-infected patient in 1986, shortly after she graduated from nursing school:

> He was young, twenty-five, and I was really new on the floor and he tried so hard to help himself. He had such horrible edema; his scrotum was so enlarged that he actually had to hold it when he got out of bed, and every day he would just get bigger and bigger, just filling up with fluids, and having massive diarrhea, and really having a very, very hard time. But he was quite alert and was conscious of everything. He was aware. I'll never forget this, one day I was with him, and he was so bloated and having such terrible diarrhea, and he really wanted to go to the commode. I got the commode, he got up, there was an explosion. It was all over everything: him, me, the floor. He was so big, and he put himself down on the bed, and he said, "I'm sorry." I was so angry at the disease. I was just so angry. It was just such a damned, horrible thing for this poor guy.

Since those early days, HIV-infected patients have become anything but a rarity, and some of the shock at the manifestations of the disease has worn off for those involved in their care. But the pity remains. Bob G., a clinic nurse in a hospital with a largely young and immigrant population of HIV patients, described it thus: "They're young. They look like us. They don't seem any different, but they don't have much time. That's what really gets you."

It is pity for the beautiful young woman on her first visit to the HIV clinic. It is pity for the IV drug users who never expected to live very long anyway, but who never expected to die this way. It is pity for the women who will never see their children as adults and for the children who die before they know what life is about. It is pity for those who lose their lovers to HIV disease and then wait to join them. It is pity and sorrow for those who could not know the consequences of the choices they made. As Alice D. said of one of her earliest patients:

> Almost all of our patients were gay men and then along came a sprinkling of women. As a matter of fact one of our first [HIV-infected] patients was a woman and I'll never forget her as long as I live. She was from ———, and I guess she had heard from her doctor that the doctor I worked with was interested in this particular problem and had a lot of experience, such as it was in that early stage of the disease. Anyway, she was a black secretary, very well educated, a lovely, lovely woman, in her mid-twenties. She was married to a man who had used drugs. At that time we didn't know what was going on; we didn't know any of the connections. She had a daughter who was five years old, and after the mother was diagnosed, of course she was worried about her daughter. So I remember we drew her [the daughter's] blood. Ordinarily we didn't care for children, but we tested her. There was no test for HIV, but we tested her T-cells, that's all we could do at the time. And she was okay. But when the mother got sick, her husband left her because he was afraid he would become infected. The irony is, in retrospect, he gave it to her, but he wasn't sick and she was. He left her so he wouldn't get sick.

Choices made before the disease was known could bring in their wake not only death but abandonment. To die is bad enough, but to be left to die is an added injury. Perhaps this scenario evokes the strongest feelings of pity and compassion. As Alice D. continued:

> Our second woman patient was a prostitute. She was from another state, and again her doctor had heard that we were interested in this particular problem, so she came over. The doctor was getting a [medical] history and this patient told us how many [sexual] contacts she had. It was some amazing number, but only for nine months of the year. The doctor asked, "Why only for nine months?" And she said, "Well, I'm a student, I'm a chemistry major at ———." That's how she worked her way through college. In the summer, I don't know if she went back home, she was from the Midwest, a very blond, scrubbed farm girl, but she worked as a prostitute for nine months of the year to work her way through college. Anyway, she had all these symptoms that I had never seen. She had all these sores on her lips, and she had herpes and other diseases, some opportunistic infections as well. She had a boyfriend who was not a pimp. She had a private life that was separate from her professional life. But he left her when she got sick. She was a nice person, too. I can't imagine why

she did what she did. I can't identify with what motivates someone to choose that lifestyle, but, of course, she had no idea how dangerous it was at the time. So she died too. And one by one, we lost them.

Choosing to Care

Compassion for the suffering of people infected with HIV and a desire to help are the first reasons most of the nurses in this study gave for their decision to become involved in the care of HIV patients. The desire to help sometimes springs from family background. Jean C., a home-care nurse, attributed her commitment to the training her parents gave her:

> My family is all in social services. My father is a policeman; my brother is a district office manager for a child welfare agency. My parents are very socially conscious, so I guess there's a strain of service there. I think there probably was. I'm not so sure I would ever have chosen accounting even if I had been given the opportunity: it just wasn't the way I was enculturated. My parents taught us that people were important, and that I needed to think of them as well as myself, and even sometimes before myself. I think that probably made a difference.

Some nurses felt compelled to become involved. Abby G. said: "When I'm in the middle of it, it's almost I feel I have to do it. And while I complain a lot about it, I don't know that I could do anything different." Carey M. agreed. She sought out her present position when she finished her MPH [master's in public health] degree.

> People say, "How can you work there?" and I say, "How can I have the education and the knowledge that I have, and the experience that I have, and not bring it to this horrendous epidemic which is going on here?" I couldn't think of not doing it. I have experience in maternal health [she worked in a HIV prenatal clinic], I have experience in addictions, and I have my master's in public health. I'm a perfect set up for it, and I couldn't not do it. I couldn't not do it.

Some nurses feel a close connection to the patients they care for; some see their work as an expression of their solidarity with those with whom they identify. A black nurse in a city hospital, said simply: "These are my people. It's my community. I want to take care of them."

This community may be a racial, ethnic, or sexual group. For some homosexuals, the appearance of the epidemic in the gay community prompted them to go into health care. One male nurse said his decision to go to nursing school coincided with the appearance of HIV disease. He went through his training with the goal of finding a job in HIV care as soon as he graduated. A lesbian nurse said her involvement with HIV-infected patients was due to her desire to help the gay community. Arthur R., another gay nurse, said he became interested in HIV disease when he worked in an emergency room and saw how the gay patients were treated. He said:

> I always felt a special bond to anyone who came in in a dress who happened to be a male, and years ago, maybe five years ago, when this thing about AIDS was coming out, no one would go near them. But I would go near them, and I felt a responsibility to them and an affinity to them. I thought it could be me. I made sure they got a good deal. If their bed needed changing, I changed their bed and all that stuff.

Other nurses simply ascribed their involvement to their ongoing commitment to providing health care, particularly to those groups not ordinarily well served by the health-care system. One nurse in an "elite" hospital said she had always nursed on the margins, in prisons and with TB patients. Now it was HIV disease. Paula T., at a city hospital, said the same thing:

> I've always worked in areas that have not been fashionable as far as nursing goes. I've worked with drug addicts, battered women, and in areas that usually people find taxing, but I've always felt that people who need the health care most are often the ones who don't get it, so I've always gravitated toward areas that people aren't clamoring to work in.

This same nurse saw herself in her patients, although on almost any kind of social scale she would seem to have little in common with them. Her patient population is predominantly IVDUs. But, as she said:

> I'm a child of the sixties, and I experimented with a lot of chemicals when I was in college, so I have a slightly different perspective on what drug abuse is. For me, it was a period of experimentation, but there were certainly enough of my peers who got lost in the whole drug experimentation period. It became a very fine line for me between who can experiment and leave it and who can't. When I began to see it as such, I really began to see it as just something that people get involved in because of who they are. And if they lose their

life to it, which I think a lot of people have actually done, it's only probably because they have no control over it, physically or emotionally. My feeling has always been, and maybe that's the way I grew up, that it could be me there, it could be someone I care about, it could be someone that I'm intimately involved with.

A significant number of these nurses have encountered HIV disease in their own lives. This can be another motivating factor in their decision to care for HIV-infected patients. Some have lost friends and family members to the disease. Lore H. feared for her brother and decided to learn as much as she could about the disease:

> AIDS has hit me both on a professional level and on a personal level. I have a brother who is HIV-infected. I had a feeling, since the statistics were that about 75 percent of gay men were infected, somehow I knew that, sooner or later, I felt that my brother was at high risk, and that he was going to come up positive, so that's what actually got me very interested in the disease.

Abby G. cared for a friend's husband and was drawn professionally into HIV care through that experience. She said:

> I was taking care of a good friend's husband who died at home, of AIDS, not on any other basis than that he was a friend of mine, and I just really got involved in treatments and the devastation it really wreaks on a family. Perhaps it's just that I always knew I had a tolerance for dealing with those kinds of things; I don't know where it comes from, but I do. I always felt that there I would be most useful. And so that's just sort of how I fell into it. And since I have a background with drug abusers, and because a large number of people with AIDS now are drug abusers, that helps as well. It sort of seemed like a natural progression.

Not all the nurses in this study have had personal brushes with HIV disease, however, and for some, their involvement comes not from personal identification with the patient or the disease, but from their professional training. They are nurses, and as nurses they are there to take care of patients. Marcia B. dates her commitment to HIV care from the early days of the epidemic when patients were openly shunned and isolated. This seemed wrong. As she said:

> I remember one patient who was an artist, and it was still at the point where everyone was wearing space suits to go into rooms. I loved to

> go to see ———, because when the place was crazy outside, I could go into his room and sit down and watch him paint. I developed a rapport that way, plus I guess it was the advocacy role that made me more involved—because of this incredible fear that was going on, from the housekeepers and nurses and doctors and everybody else. Because, back then, patients would say, "Why do people come in dressed like that, the gowns, the masks, the gloves?" I had some housekeepers who put on hats and booties just to walk in the door, not to go near the patient, just to mop or to empty the garbage, and they wouldn't speak to patients. They probably wouldn't even look. But I guess, early on, I had two or three patients who were there two or three months, and who repeated, and I developed a relationship with them, so they became very important, the same as any patient I had for three or four months, and I resented it when people upset them. So it was an advocacy role. I think that's how the interest developed. That goes back to my undergraduate education. I was taught from day one "You are the patient's advocate."

Emma J., a nurse clinician at a suburban hospital, was similarly propelled into HIV care when she discovered that many of her colleagues felt justified in refusing to care for HIV-infected patients. As she described her path to HIV care:

> When I first started reading about AIDS, I was interested. Something drew me. I wanted to know what was going on. I was working at a blood service at the time, and I missed bedside nursing. I loved bedside nursing, but I took the blood service job because it was a day job. I had been working nights, and I couldn't do that any more. But I always missed the hospital, and I started reading about AIDS, and I started reading about nurses and doctors who wouldn't take care of these patients. I couldn't understand it at all. And a nurse I know told me about the refresher course for nurses she was taking, and how they spent a day on HIV, what it entails and all that sort of thing, psychological aspects and whatever. The students in the course were asked to go home and talk to their families about it and come back the next day and tell the instructor how they felt about taking care of AIDS patients. So they all came back and said, "No way, never." I was infuriated. Absolutely infuriated. I said, "Okay, that's it. Put your money where your mouth is." So I went to a seminar and then started working at ———.

Nina H. had a similar reaction to the way the first HIV-infected patient on her floor was treated:

> My first patient here [in a city hospital] was really ignored. I wasn't aware exactly of what she had then, but I still remember I was not happy with how she was being treated. It wasn't any blatant abuse, but it was very subtle things like keeping her door closed all the time. She wound up bleeding out and dying, and I remember they kept closing the door. The head nurse, when I went to talk to her about it, told me not to get too close. . . . On another floor, we had a few patients with AIDS, and I'd watch the aides go in to bring a glass of juice or something wearing everything. If they weren't wearing gowns, gloves, masks, the works, they would not go in to see if the patient was okay. I watched one nurse in a room which had an observation window. She banged on the door and the patient took his temperature and then held up the thermometer at the window so she could read it and did not have to go in. That bothered me.

Sometimes the appeal of this work comes from the opportunity to set up something new, to be in at the start and establish a program to take care of HIV-infected patients. Because HIV disease prompts such strong negative reactions from many health-care professionals, some hospitals have opted for dedicated AIDS units where all the patients have been definitively diagnosed as HIV-infected or suffering from AIDS. For those able and interested in taking care of HIV-infected patients, these units offer fine opportunities. Gladys R. said that this kind of opportunity was part of what drew her to HIV care, much as it had drawn her to other areas of nursing:

> As long as I've been working now, maybe about thirty years, I like to be where there's something new, where there's a challenge. When they first started dialysis, I opened the dialysis unit, and when I came here, they started IV therapy, and now I'm head of the IV therapy in the AIDS unit. Where there is somewhere where I can make a start, a start from the bottom up, and see it grow, that's a challenge. I like a challenge like that. About five or six years down the road, it becomes a little bit too commonplace. You're just there, nothing to really challenge you, and I'm ready to go.

Part of what also attracted Gladys was the chance to do the job right. She had been upset when nurses in other units of the hospital wanted no part of HIV care. She said that, by joining the new unit dedicated to HIV-infected patients,

> we were going to let the patients know that we weren't afraid of them, so we only wore gloves when we had to do things with their

> blood, and their feces and urine and things like that. Otherwise, with patient contact, we didn't wear gowns and gloves or masks. We wore masks only if it was a respiratory isolation, or we wore gloves if making skin contact and if they had sores or wounds or things like that. This was the first time this was being done, because in other places they had to put on the gowns and masks and boots, and they would take the tray and slide it in the room. Our [unit] was going to be a pilot. We touched the patient and rubbed their backs and things like that. This was the way we opened up.

Commitment to caring for patients with HIV disease thus comes from a number of directions: from personal values, from professional training, from identification with the patient. It can also flow from an intellectual interest in the disease itself. HIV disease is intriguing. It has myriad manifestations. As Alicia P., a staff nurse in a voluntary hospital, said:

> You never know what system is going to be affected. For example, if you had someone with leukemia, you know where you'd have to look; like, if their platelet count is very low, you don't want to give them intramuscular injections. So you know what to assess and what to look for. But in this every organ system is involved: their skin, their nervous system, orthopedic problems, their lungs, their heart, eye infections. It's every organ system you have to monitor.

In order to provide the care needed, a nurse has to stay on top of developments and keep abreast of what's happening. This can be intellectually challenging and satisfying. Alicia went on to say:

> You really have to be on top of the things you have to know. One drug may give them seizures. When we gave pentamidine in the early days, instead of inhaling it we used to give it intravenously, and it would make their blood sugar go way down, and they'd get hypoglycemic. It's the whole gamut. You're not just dealing with a forty-year-old guy who had a heart attack. You're dealing with a lot of complex issues.

This is part of what makes caring for patients with HIV disease attractive. It is an opportunity to be involved in something new and challenging, something which demands concentration and attention. Gloria R., a midwife who has practiced for twenty years and whose position—before her present one in an HIV prenatal clinic—involved developing programs to prevent premature births, attributed part of her interest in HIV care to the challenge of bringing HIV-infected women to term and through delivery:

> I like doing high-risk pregnancy. I mean I never would have thought a few years back that I would be doing this or doing the prevention of prematurity. I loved doing regular prenatal and deliveries, but I also like the challenge of high-risk. I liked the women I was taking care of in the prematurity study who had had previous stillborns or second trimester losses; there was intense follow-up with those women, and I liked that. I would never say that regular pregnancy or delivery are boring, because they aren't, but this [caring for HIV-infected pregnant women] is a little bit more challenging to me, and I like that. I like that.

Part of the appeal of caring for HIV-infected patients can be the pleasure of working with dynamic and caring colleagues. Many nurses remarked that one of the satisfactions of HIV care was working with like-minded staff. Gloria R. was attracted to HIV care partly because she liked the woman who recruited her:

> The project manager [for this position] came to our chapter meeting to talk about this program she was setting up and said that they were looking for nurses. So I'm sitting in this meeting and I said to myself, "I like this woman." She was about my age, very laid back, and I could see she was honest and caring. So I said, "Give me your card and I'll call you tomorrow." So we talked on the telephone and we set up an appointment and it was just like love at first sight. I knew that I wanted to work with this woman because I could see that she was really into it and dedicated to it. She wasn't doing it because it was a job; in fact all the people in the program, the people who work here, choose to work here because they're interested to work here and they want to help, and I got the sense that they were really caring and it wasn't just a study. They got the grant and they worked it all out, but they weren't just doing it because "Oh yeah, here's a grant, we'll do a grant," but their heart is in it.

This is one of the reasons many nurses prefer to work in all-HIV units. A special inpatient or outpatient unit for HIV-infected patients or a residential facility for long-term care of AIDS patients offers nurses the support of colleagues whose values and practice match their own. This is particularly important in HIV care, because the disease and the patients it infects inspire fear and avoidance among health personnel. Many of the nurses in this study reported that they were stigmatized, questioned, and/or ridiculed by other health-care workers because they cared for HIV-infected patients. It can be difficult to maintain one's convictions when colleagues think otherwise. As Peter Berger comments, "Most of what we 'know' we have taken on the authority of others, and it is only as others continue to confirm this 'knowledge' that it continues to be plausible to us" (1990 [1969]: 7).

Nurses caring for HIV-infected patients need confirmation that they are doing the right thing, that these patients have a right to care, and that nursing intervention can mitigate the terrors of the disease. Nurses in HIV care can suffer a kind of siege mentality, because the stigma of the disease and the fear it engenders, even for those who have chosen to do this kind of nursing, can cut them off from their friends, families, and colleagues. The nurses may become stigmatized themselves. A dedicated HIV unit, therefore, can provide cognitive and emotional support and encouragement. Working in a group committed to caring for HIV-infected patients eliminates some of the stress of continually having to justify, either to oneself or one's coworkers, the correctness of one's behavior. As Robin M. said:

> In general what I like is the motivation of the other health-care workers in AIDS. I work with people who have also chosen to work with AIDS. If you go to other units, you will find AIDS patients there but the nurses, doctors, and other caretakers have not really chosen to work with AIDS. Sometimes I see reluctance, and sometimes I even see hostility, towards me or towards the patient, which is worse, even if it's latent. They won't say, "Well, I hate you because you use drugs," but there is that little undertone that I sense. And here [in a dedicated AIDS unit] I come in and I feel like I'm coming home. Here people really look out for the patients. They say, "Oh, I went into Joe's room and he's doing so much better and I brought him some chili. He likes chili." Or, "I'm going out to Wendy's, what should I bring Mary?" They buy for the patients. They pay for the TV. It's a crowd that wants to work here, and that's very important. I like to associate with the group that's interested in AIDS care.

It is also true that for some of these nurses HIV care has given them professional opportunities otherwise not often available in nursing. Many nurses cited the job itself as an inducement to specialize in HIV care. Along with commitment to care and concern for the patient as well as interest in the disease, there comes to these women and men a realization that HIV offers the kinds of jobs they have been searching for. In the United States, nursing has always felt hampered by its beginnings, first as a domestic responsibility of women and then as an adjunct to scientific medicine (Reverby 1987; Melosh 1982). Professional nursing is still seeking a way to stand alone.

HIV disease offers some nurses the opportunity to practice autonomously and to achieve an independent status. Most nurses said that their autonomy was greater in HIV care than in other specialties, and the majority reported that they experienced improved collaboration and collegiality with physicians. Because physicians are not flocking to take care of patients with HIV disease, some institutions are turning to nurses to provide primary health care. In one hospital, the HIV unit is under the daily supervision of a nurse practitioner, not a doctor. One of the nurse practitioners in my sample accepted a fellowship in primary HIV care offered by a leading voluntary hospital. These positions have a great deal of responsibility. Carol H., a nurse practitioner in a residential facility, described her position:

> It's really the best job I've ever had. I like the autonomy. I like very much not being part of a structured [work setting]. I never liked working in a hospital. I did inpatient on the floor for only about six months, and that was right after I graduated from nursing school, and the rest of the time it's been public health nursing or working as a nurse practitioner in a health clinic. I put in more than the number of hours required, but nobody checks on them, and it's just very gratifying. I'm pretty much on call twenty-four hours a day, but that's okay.

Lena F., whose colleagues pointed out to her that without HIV she wouldn't have her job, replied that she didn't want anyone to be sick, she didn't want to see anyone suffer, but at the same time, she said:

> This is one of the most gratifying jobs I could have as a nurse, because I feel I'm using every skill that I have, that I've been taught, that I've acquired over the years. I really think I'm doing as much as I can; I'm working to capacity. I'm really able to give. I'm not just going in and saying, "Well, I have three baths to give, and I have to give out twenty meds, and the patient doesn't want to hear what meds." Here the patients really listen to me, they give me respect, they listen, they value my opinions. It's a very interactive process.

The desire to use their skills and talents to the fullest is another reason many of these nurses cited for their decision to become involved in HIV care. They are proud of what they can do for patients. They find that they can alleviate their patients' suffering, whether the suffering comes from physical, intellectual or emotional distress. That they can respond in so many different ways and that they know what can be done and how to do it is a source of great satisfaction.

To be successful at caring for HIV-infected patients, nurses have to draw on all their capacities and be willing to continue to learn. It requires commitment and dedication. On AIDS units, nurses' development is facilitated by a lower than usual nurse/patient ratio. Nurses have more time per patient and can care for their patients at a comfortable pace.

One municipal hospital opened its HIV unit with ten patients and five nurses. It has since failed to maintain that ratio, but its record in this area is still far better than on other units where, in this particular hospital, there can be one registered nurse for forty patients during the day and none at night. Most AIDS units have between five and eight patients per nurse. This desirable nurse-patient ratio has been used as a recruiting inducement by some HIV units, but it alone cannot attract nurses. In the municipal hospital mentioned above, it is still difficult to attract nurses to the HIV unit, even though nurses on the regular wards may already be caring for as many or more HIV-infected patients as the dedicated unit.

If working conditions alone determined nurses' decisions, dedicated HIV units would be flooded with applicants. Some units do have waiting lists, but these are well-run units with a demonstrable esprit de corps. Not all staff on HIV units work well, even when staffed with nurses committed to HIV-infected patients. The human mix is always an important factor.

None of the nurses with whom I spoke cited just one reason for becoming involved with HIV care. Most mentioned the desire to help first, but with all of them there were also issues of personal development and professional growth. There is no one profile that fits these nurses. Some find that they want to be by the bedside; others can't get away from it fast enough. Some like hospitals; some prefer home care. Some focus on managing the symptoms of the disease; some are more interested in the psychosocial aspects. Some gravitate toward taking care of women and children; others prefer IV drug users. Still others find homosexual patients the most satisfying to work with. The variety of the manifestations of this disease offers nurses a number of different ways of being involved. There are different practice settings, different patient populations, different symptoms. Each has its particular challenges and satisfactions.

The different groups who are infected with HIV, the different infections and conditions they suffer, the various settings within which care is given—these make it possible for nurses who want to care for HIV-infected patients to be involved with the kinds of patients they feel most drawn to, in the setting in which they feel most comfortable. Those who work best with highly educated and motivated middle-class patients are able to work with them. Those who find the greatest satisfaction working with groups on the margins of society or those actively rejected by society have no trouble finding them. Nurses who want to care for gays or for women and children or for black or Hispanic groups are sure to locate opportunities.

Nurses who like the support of institutional structures gravitate toward hospital work. Nurses who like to be on their own, perhaps more intimately involved with patients in informal settings, will choose home care. Nurses who like research can find positions in clinical trials. Nurses who want direct patient contact can find it in different intensities in hospitals and clinics and home care. Nurses who want a more distant role may also find a number of positions in administration or teaching. Just as there is no one model of HIV disease, so there is no one model of HIV nursing.

Until very recently the nursing shortage, coupled with increasing demand for nursing care, gave nurses in New York City unparalleled job opportunities. When I started my research in 1989, an administrator told me that the demand for personnel was so great that any nurse at a municipal hospital could walk out and get a job at a more prestigious institution. And indeed as the "elite" voluntary hospitals, whose patients are usually well-heeled or well-insured, opened HIV units in the late eighties, they often recruited nurses who had experience with HIV from city hospitals.

Because of the nurse shortage, salaries for nurses increased substantially in the late 1980s, to the point where staff nurses with twenty or more years of experience could command $60,000 to $70,000 in elite hospitals, with substantial additions from overtime. It is now not unheard of for a head nurse in an elite hospital to make close to $100,000 a year. New graduates in voluntary hospitals now start with a base salary of $40,000 with differentials for night duty and/or specialty positions. Municipal hospitals pay about ten percent less. Positions beyond the staff nurse level pay higher salaries in all hospitals, and there is an additional increment for advanced degrees.

These numbers are, of course, gratifying to a profession that has been traditionally underpaid, but the nurses in this study were working and continued to work when salaries were much lower. In 1987 one member of the sample, a nurse with a master's degree, accepted a staff position in a voluntary hospital at a salary of $26,000. Another said her salary in 1983, as a staff nurse in a dedicated AIDS unit in a municipal hospital, was $23,000.

But there is no doubt that the nurses I interviewed took advantage of the demand for nurses to find the jobs they wanted. This is an attractive aspect of the profession of nursing. As Nina H. said:

> You have to go into it with wide-open eyes and understand that you're not going to be rich and famous. You're not. But I am so glad to be doing what I'm doing. One of the reasons I went into nursing was the amount of choice within the field. One of my friends from nursing school is in obstetrics; another is in a doctor's office. Another guy I went to school with runs a cardiac catheter lab. There's a host of things to go into. You can do administration, or teaching, or occupational nursing, public health. The possibilities are endless. What other field has this range of choices? Even with the minimum degree, the R.N., you can go far.

Among the nurses in the Association of Nurses in AIDS Care (ANAC), there is a continual sharing of information about jobs and opportunities. In order to take advantage of these opportunities, nurses have to keep current. Sometimes they have to take a refresher course, and they have to take the initiative. But there are so many different kinds of positions for nurses that savvy practitioners have a luxury of choice unknown to many other professionals.

The arrival of HIV disease in the 1980s opened up a number of new nurse positions in the New York City health-care system. At a time when hospital beds, system-wide, were being eliminated, the AIDS epidemic provided a growth sector in the health industry. New units, new clinics, new home-care agencies were opened. Each of these offered nurses the chance to move, if they were willing to develop an expertise in HIV disease.

Chapter 4
Empathy and Challenge

When the trickle of patients with HIV disease turned into a stream and then a torrent, it became apparent that the incidence of the disease varied geographically and demographically. The first to be significantly threatened were young, white, gay men living in large cities. The homosexual communities in New York and San Francisco were hardest hit. Intravenous drug users were the second group to be affected. Again, they tended to cluster in large cities where drug use was endemic. Numbers of young, black and Hispanic men, predominantly IVDUs, though some were also gay, began to appear in hospital units, clinics, and as referrals to home-care agencies. The third group, currently the fastest growing (though numerically still far fewer than gay men or IVDUs), is that of women and children. Women contract HIV disease most often through their own drug use; the second largest number of women become HIV-infected because their sex partner is infected.

There are also, of course, patients who have HIV disease but who do not fit the categories of homosexual or bisexual, drug user, or partner of a homosexual, bisexual, or drug user. Their numbers, however, are very small.

From several points of view, PWAs have from the start been unsettling to those charged with the responsibility to care for them. Not only was their disease a mystery, but they themselves were new to the health-care system. Until HIV disease appeared, both gay men and IVDUs avoided mainstream care. Then HIV disease brought both groups into extensive contact with the mainstream health-care system. Quite suddenly, beginning in 1981, large numbers of gay men and IVDUs began to come for care at both public and private hospitals.

Most of the nurses in this study were not familiar with these kinds of patients at the start of the 1980s, and in order to understand their special characteristics, the nurses needed to call on their professional commitments and their personal skills. Their professional training made clear that these people were something other than the sum of their social characteristics; when they came for care, they were "patients."

Patients are simply people in distress, in need of care, care which a nurse knows how to provide. The category of "patient" enables the nurse to leave aside the particularities that social labels such as gay or IVDU suggest in order to focus instead on the individual as a person in need of care. The person's social characteristics have an impact on care—they must be taken into account—but they ought not, in this construction, disturb the basic posture of nurse and patient. The nurse proffers help, and the patient accepts it. Yet the generalizing and abstracting effect of the concept of "patient" has to mesh with an understanding of social characteristics if care is going to be appropriate to the individual. It is here that nurses begin to use personal skills of empathy and engagement, because it is essential to bridge the gap between themselves and their patients if they are to provide proper care.

The essence of these nurses' approach to their patients is acceptance of the "other." Ideally, they do not judge; instead they seek to understand. Although their own personal convictions and codes of behavior may be very different from those of their patients, such differences are not allowed to interfere with the process of understanding. Off duty, these nurses might be critical or despairing of their patients. But on duty, their mental attitude is one of receptivity and acceptance.

Some nurses in this study contrasted their own attitudes with those of colleagues who had difficulty caring for gay men or IVDUs. They told me of older nurses, and those trained in other countries, who were sometimes totally unprepared for the kinds of patients for whom they were asked to care. Nina H., a young nurse in a municipal hospital, commented:

> There are older nurses here, and to ask a fifty-five-year-old woman to deal with a transsexual who's a cross dresser, for example, is a lot. We've had some real blatant queens, the ones who have already had the breast implants and stuff, and some of the nurses here are really shocked.

Some of the nurses who have trouble caring for PWAs are uncomfortable because they disapprove of the patient's behavior on moral grounds; others are simply embarrassed to bring up sexuality or drug abuse, even though knowing whether the patient engages in these activities is important in planning care. Whole areas of life that used to be matters of only private concern are being brought out into the open with HIV disease (Gee 1989).

In addition, even for nurses who have worked for years in the municipal hospital system, the HIV-infected population can be distressing because so many patients are so very poor and so very needy in so many different ways. There have always been "service patients," patients whose care is paid for with public funds. But even in municipal hospitals these patients were interspersed among middle-class and working-class patients. With HIV disease, the patient population is becoming increasingly poor and marginalized. It is a group without much of a toehold in mainstream America. This can be upsetting to nurses who, through their profession, have achieved middle-class standing and who value middle-class standards.

The changes in patient population from gay, white males to IVDU males to IVDU women and the partners of IVDU males makes nursing itself more challenging; teaching and counseling about good health habits and medication schedules have to be geared to the patient's capacities. Nurses cannot assume, with the most recently infected patient populations, that their patients lead well-regulated lives and that they possess the skills needed to comply with complex medical regimens. One nurse said:

> It never really bothered me [that patients wouldn't keep appointments, etc.] because I did my master's thesis on why the poor didn't avail themselves of health care. In the course of doing that I think I learned a lot about what it's like to be poor. Also, my previous experience at the home-care agency taught me a lot about why people act the way they do. So I think I have become more tolerant of things than maybe some of the younger nurses who haven't been exposed to so much or come from a wholly different environment. I have a background where I never had a fear of patients or where they lived. It never really bothered me. So part of what I do is work with the younger nurses and help them understand why some people do the things they do.

But some of the nurses I interviewed said they had to work at developing the openness they needed. Even nurses fully committed to HIV care can be uncomfortable talking about sexuality or drug use. It is not unusual for patients to ask nurses about the safety of oral and anal sex. Suzette J., in charge of education at a city hospital, grew up in a very liberal European country, but even she had to learn a lot before she felt comfortable dealing with certain subjects.

> I don't have a problem now talking about sex or a problem talking about needles. I used to have, but I learned not to be embarrassed, because otherwise I might as well sit behind my desk and not get up. We're not going to change anything if we don't know about drugs or sex, or when we ourselves are uncomfortable talking about them. Many, many people are. I'm not anymore and some of the patients look at me very surprised, thinking, "Here she comes in her middle-class way, and she talks about shooting up, and uses terms we use on the streets." I think it helps that I can talk freely about such things.

Nina H., who worked in the same hospital as Suzette, agreed:

> I feel that anyone who works in HIV should have at least one course in sexuality. If you're not comfortable saying the words or the terms, there is no way you can counsel somebody. I've had discussions with people about whether blow jobs can transmit AIDS, and sometimes they don't know how to say it. I'll have to say, "going down" or "blow job." So you have to be comfortable hearing it and saying it.

Central to the acceptance the nurses in this study practice is the ability to put their own preferences and beliefs aside. These nurses do not bring their own code into the workplace, although several told me that they heard many things that shocked them and many things that they would rather not have known. As Nina H. went on to say:

> I had one woman tell me how she gave blow jobs to pay her rent. I can't judge her, but it's not what I would like to do, and I really felt like telling her, "Don't you feel like you're being used?" But it was an uncomfortable situation for her, and I wasn't going to make it worse.

It can work the other way, too, when nurses' attitudes are more liberal than their patient's. Marcia B., working in a municipal hospital where every kind of ethnic and racial group was represented, said of one of her AIDS patients:

> I had a patient who was Muslim, and he felt that God was punishing him for his homosexuality. So I had to be careful talking around that. It wasn't a matter of not saying anything. I had to appreciate that, for someone like him, I had to let him denigrate himself. He had to express his feelings. He understood that it was the virus, but he took AIDS as punishment, and at this point I'm not going to make him comfortable about his homosexuality. There's no way he's going to change his thinking. And it's not for me to become a sex therapist.

The ability to distinguish between what one would do oneself and what one's patients do is critical to providing good care. Instead of one's own values, others' standards come into play. In such a situation, the nurse tries to think and feel as the patient might think and feel. This has been called "negative capability." It means entering another's world. To do this, the nurse must understand the patient's "culture," the thoughts, habits, practices, prejudices, pleasures, and pains that the patient takes for granted but that the nurse may not. As Cassie N., a staff nurse in a voluntary hospital where most of the patients were gay, explained:

> On the average floor, you might get a little uncomfortable with a husband getting into bed with his wife during her hospitalization. Well, here, you deal with that, but it might be two males. And as long as they're not disturbing a roommate, or doing something flagrant, or doing something that's going to make them worse, there isn't any reason why people shouldn't show affection. You just have to learn to get past that strange feeling. Some people get over it very quickly. Some people, it takes a while.

Accepting the patient is the first step in the process of discovery for these nurses. Nina H. said of her patients:

> Here in ——— [a city hospital], the majority of patients are IVDUs; they're homeless, they have no support systems. A lot of them are still actively using drugs, even on the wards. That's the majority. So you're really dealing with a difficult personality to start. They don't trust the system, the whole system. They are not used to the system in terms of actually being able to get something from it. And you're dealing with sick people. They've been through so much. Just look at their histories. Think of a patient who's had surgery for gunshots, stabbings. He's been in and out of jail. He's been living in a men's shelter for six years, and he's thirty, an alcoholic. Now he has AIDS. It's a life I can't fathom. But I realize that I'm dealing with a population that's very different from me, disenfranchised and so on. And a different race and different ethnicity. That's a given in any city hospital. Everyone here has to want to get over it [the difference]. It's one of the things that keeps me here.

After bridging the differences, the next step for nurses is using what they discover to reach and teach the patient. These nurses, for example, have learned how to phrase questions properly to get the information they need. Many of their IVDU patients come from Central and

South America, so the nurses need to become literate in those patients' cultural concepts. This means, among other things, knowing how sex is conceptualized in other ethnic groups. Marcia B. noted that Hispanic men do not think about sex between men in the same way that Americans do. She said:

> Very often South American men, all the different countries, they don't think of themselves as homosexual. And if you ask them, they'll say, "No." But if you say, "Have you had sex with a man?" they'll say, "Yes." But you can't say, "Are you gay?" "Are you a homosexual?" They'll say, "No."

Nurses' do not always find their own openness and ability to discuss sexuality and drug use reflected in their patients. Marcia B. went on to say that "the women, a lot of times, will not want to tell on the male, so they'll deny all risk factors. I still think of one woman, up to the day she died, she denied. And you knew the husband was a shooter, you just knew." One nurse who is Hispanic, and whose patients are Hispanic, remarked that sex is not commonly talked about in the homes of her patients, and so trying to talk about safe sex, particularly with the men, is a challenge. She said of one patient, "He won't even look at me. He puts his head down. So I just keep talking, and leave the condoms, and hope that he's absorbing some of it." In such a situation, the nurse has to find a way to make her meaning clear to her patient without criticizing his beliefs and values.

This same nurse started postpartum classes for Hispanic women at her hospital, classes where they could discuss birth control and other issues related to sexuality. But, she said, her patients did not feel at risk. It is hard to convince people that they are in danger if they are feeling well. And advice about the use of condoms can run counter to fiercely held beliefs about who decides what between men and women.

One patient who went home and suggested to her partner that he use condoms returned to the clinic with a black eye. The nurse who had made the recommendation felt responsible for her patient's injury. At the time I talked to her, she was puzzling out how to change and tailor her educational program to her patient's situation. The advice she was giving was medically accurate but socially disastrous. She was looking for a way to bring the two realms into alignment. She had not found the solution at the time of our interview, and yet in her response one can see the contours of the kind of thinking that makes it possible for these nurses to understand their patients' worlds.

What they come to understand they then use to improve the care patients receive. They incorporate what they learn into practice. As Stephanie C. said:

> There are adolescents in the community who don't like to use condoms, and they're sexually active. Also, among the Hispanic community, they tend to use anal intercourse to preserve the virginity of the girl. For young girls, virginity is prized. When I learned this, I said, "Oh, my God," because this increases her risk. And she may be a virgin, but she may have AIDS. She may not get pregnant, but she may get AIDS. So, when we do sexual counseling with these girls, when we do a sexual interview with them, and the doctor asks them, "Have you had intercourse?" she'll say, "No," because they mean vaginal intercourse. She'll say, "I'm a virgin." And the doctor doesn't go any further. So we have to tell doctors how to do a proper sexual history.

The nurses in this study tried to look without preconceptions and moral judgments at how their patients lived. This enabled them not only to understand their patients but to present their patients' concerns and values to others in a sympathetic manner. Because nurses occupy a position where several worlds come together, many of the nurses in this study felt responsible for changing the perceptions of other health-care workers who were unable or reluctant to put themselves in the HIV patient's place. Emily D., who moved from direct bedside care of HIV-infected patients to teaching licensed practical nurses in a home-care agency, said of her work:

> We're constantly having to educate people about the person's sexual orientation as part of their life. I tell them "Maybe you're uncomfortable asking that question, but you have to; you have to know." I had one nurse say to me that the patient was all upset because his roommate just died, and I said, "Was it his roommate or his lover?" She was embarrassed to ask. And I said, "Look, there's a big difference between losing your roommate and losing your lover." So that kind of thing comes up. With IVDUs, a lot of the nurses don't want to deal with the issue, so they don't even ask if they're doing drugs any more. And I have to be constantly pointing out to them that not only do you have to worry about symptoms but, also, are they sharing needles? Are they keeping their needles clean? Are they sexually active? It's interesting how some people will put on their blinders, and they'll focus on the disease, and then they'll just ignore these things over here, all the social characteristics and the stuff that makes them uncomfortable.

Not ignoring "all that stuff" is what makes these nurses effective, because it may be exactly that which one needs to know to decide what to do for a patient. As the nurse quoted above explained:

> Say I go in, and I find a patient who's acting a little strange, whose mental status is a little off, and I'm trying to decide, "Did he just get high or does he have a central nervous system infection?" I had this situation when I was doing home care. So I asked him, "Did you just shoot up? I need to know whether to call the doctor." And he said, "Yeah." So I said, "What did you do?" In this case, he had shot heroin and cocaine mixed together, which they call a speedball on the street, and his pulse was 150. I had just taken his pulse, and I had to say, "Tell me what you did, because otherwise I have to get an ambulance because your pulse is 150."

As this example demonstrates, it is essential that the nurse get to know the patient well, because every aspect of living can affect the progress of the disease. Getting to know the patient intimately—in greater depth and detail than the standard medical history—is therefore an integral part of these nurses' jobs.

Many of the nurses in my sample who took care of white, gay men said these were the best patients they ever encountered. They found the process of getting to know them pleasurable. On average, at the beginning of the epidemic, gay patients were middle class and well educated. Many had strong support systems of lovers and friends. They frequently knew more than their nurses about their disease. They were on top of the latest information. As Tom R., who worked in an elite hospital where almost all the patients were gay and middle class, said:

> I read everything I can get my hands on, and all of my patients bring me in articles. I tell them I don't have time to read the *New York Times* every day, so if there's anything in it, please cut it out. And they do. Mainly my patients are my main source of updating. They're the ones with the disease. They're the ones doing the research, and a lot of them do a lot of research and really keep up with the latest information. That's a change for medicine, and that's making nurses and doctors feel uncomfortable, when your patients come in asking about the newest treatment and you've never heard about it. They send for all the literature, and they read it thoroughly. They very often bring up these radical new things in meetings, and we discuss them, and pick them apart, and say what might be wrong with them, and why people don't need to jump on every bandwagon.

These gay patients often kept track of their medications and their infections. If they were hospitalized, they were able to tell their nurses just when they had their last bout of pneumonia, for example, and what treatment they had. This saves time and work for the nurse. Thus, with many gay patients, it was easy for these nurses to establish a cooperative reciprocity.

Nurse and patient often met as friends, as people who had grown fond of each other and who enriched each other's lives. Some of these patients became very special to their nurses. As Emily D. said of one such patient:

> I had this one patient, an artist; his whole apartment was just filled with things. He was a graphic artist and designer. He designed posters and bathing suits and he just loved life. He would, on his good days, he would steer the conversation into what else was happening, even though he couldn't go out anymore. But he always wanted to know, "Well, what did you do last weekend? Have you gone to any movies? Have you gone to any plays?"

As the numbers of HIV-infected patients grew, the proportion of white, gay, male HIV-infected patients dropped, and the proportion of patients who are or were IVDUs or the sexual partners of IVDUs rose. These are very different patients from the gay men who first contracted the disease. Alice D. explained what happened when her patient population changed from gay men to IV drug users:

> The patients we had who were gay men were wonderful. Most of them were well educated, middle class, hard workers, bright, funny, just great people, people you'd want to be around. And they were compliant; they wanted to help themselves. Whereas with the IVDUs, the nature of the practice changed. All of a sudden, we had to start watching where we put our money. We had to consider safety factors, security factors that we never had to before. And that's not fun. We had never been robbed, we always kept petty cash in a drawer, but we never locked the drawer, although I was running in and out of different rooms. But the first IVDU patient came in with a friend and when my head was turned, the cash disappeared. Then, later, when I worked in the AIDS unit in the hospital, we had to be careful that people weren't bringing drugs into [the unit]. We noticed that patients would sometimes leave the unit, and we found out that they were going over to another unit, meeting friends there, and shooting up. Some of their behavior was violent and abusive. It requires a lot more skills than nursing another population.

As Carol M., who worked at a hospice where most of the patients were IVDUs, explained: "Many nurses would rather work with a gay patient than with IVDUs, because a lot of the IVDUs, it's so hard to connect with them. One of the reasons they do drugs is because they don't trust easily, and they're very angry about feeling so alone. But rather than reaching out, they pull in, and they do drugs."

It is hard, in general, to establish a mutual, reciprocal, open and accessible relationship with IVDUs. As a group, they are poor, often homeless, and disconnected from society. The skills they have acquired in order to survive on the streets do not serve them well in the bureaucratic, middle-class setting of a hospital or clinic. They can be abrasive and threatening as well as charming and cajoling. Either way, they tend to believe that rules and regulations do not apply to them. In medicine and nursing, where there are detailed protocols and procedures, such an attitude breeds conflict. Gladys R. described some of her struggles with IVDU patients:

> If they know they can get [the pain medication] here, they'll carry on until they get what they want, and then they'll tell all their friends to come too. They'll tell them, "Go to ———; you can get whatever you want." Which is sometimes true. The doctors will put them on more and more to shut them up. They'll put patients on massive doses [of pain medication], even if I say, "Please cut her down or cut him down; my patient doesn't need it." I've had patients come up to me and say, "Oh, nurse, I need my medication," and I say, "Go back to your room and I'll bring it to you." When I go in their room, I find music playing and they're busy dancing. I say, "Oh, I see you're feeling much better."

IVDUs present real management problems. Their manipulative ways are legendary, and it takes a confident personality to deal with them. Everything can become a battle. Gladys R., whose unit was filled with IVDUs at the time I spoke with her, said of them:

> One thing I want to say about the IVDUs, the street people. They live in the street, they have nothing, they have nobody. They come to the hospital, they want everything and everybody to give them their full attention. They'll say, "I asked for two pork chops. How come I only got one?" Or they'll say, "My bed hasn't been changed." They'll come in and they'll be filthy, and we'll say, "We can't work with you; you need to take a bath." Lord, they fight you tooth and nail to get in the tub. Then, once they get in, you can't get them out. They're in the water; they don't want to come out. And we say, "Wait a minute,

> there's other people besides you. Wait your turn." And they come out and they tell you, "My room hasn't been cleaned yet; look at it, it's filthy." And they'll open up the air conditioner and say, "Look at that, that's why I'm coughing; the air conditioner is filthy." I mean, give me a break! They come off the street, living on the sidewalk, and now they want the Ritz!

Dealing with IVDUs takes strength of will. One nurse described patients who would stand silently in front of her desk for hours in an effort to extract additional pain medication, even though they were told to return to their rooms. Ethel G., who worked with Gladys, said:

> Oh, they curse you out. They treat you like you are their maid, not their nurse, and you have to be extremely strict with them to set limits. You have to set limits because otherwise they will run right over you. They will steal your things, anyone's things, even the outpatients' things. They even steal the other patients' food that you just left on the desk. When you come back, it's gone. So it's hard on the nurses.

Drug use continues for many patients even in the hospital. Friends bring them supplies, and the drug is commonly added to the IV bag. This happens in the very best voluntary hospitals as well as in city hospitals where close surveillance is impossible. In one hospital, the situation got so lax that patients could leave the unit, buy drugs on the street, and then come back to their rooms. The nurse who described this to me said of this situation: "They swear up and down that they never went out of the building. They take their clothes and they put them on behind the stairs. They come back, they put on their pajamas and walk in like they've never been anywhere. They claim they haven't been. They say they've been in their room watching TV or something."

This is an extreme example, but in general IVDUs can be difficult patients because they do not reciprocate. The nurse may be ready to understand but, because nursing requires a response from the patient, only half of the equation is in place if the patient does not do his part. As Ethel G. said, "You want it to be fifty-fifty. You're there to help and the patient is there to get well. Everybody should work together." This is not easy to achieve. Margaret T., the coordinator of several units for HIV-infected patients, said of the IVDU population:

> People just don't like them. They don't talk like we talk, they don't act like we act. They have no manners; they don't appreciate what's being done for them. They're obnoxious. They insult you, and

> they're demanding. I have times when I just stand and hold on because you can't give them the satisfaction of seeing you lose control, because then they have won, and it's all over. But then you can't say, "I'm not going to deal with you," and run away either.

Yet for nurses who can accept them as they are, who enjoy the challenge, who do not ask them to change beyond what they are capable of changing, IVDUs or substance abusers can be rewarding to work with. Carol M. said of them:

> Substance abusers can be delightful people. As long as your expectations are realistic, as long as you don't anticipate major changes, they are what they are. They will try to be manipulative, and you can't let your feelings get hurt and all that, but otherwise they are delightful. They make you laugh. It's rewarding to work with them.

Dealing successfully with drug addicts as patients means being able to tailor one's expectations to reality, being ready to meet them on their own ground and at their own level, and yet also continuing to work toward better health behavior.

Although the same could be said of all nursing and all patients, HIV-infected patients make unusual demands on nurses' personal skills and emotional fortitude. Almost all the nurses I interviewed said that coping with patients' emotional needs was their greatest challenge. Even middle-class patients—patients who had insurance and were not dependent on public programs and who might, therefore, be expected to be relatively self-sufficient—looked to their nurses for emotional support. As Fran L., whose patients were mostly white, gay men, said:

> If they have HIV disease and it's progressed to full-blown AIDS and they're going downhill, a lot of their support system falls by the wayside. They don't have as many people as, say, a cancer patient or a Crohn's disease patient. They may have lost some of their support system to AIDS also, so they come to rely on their home infusion and their home therapy caregivers to an unbelievable extent.

Most HIV-infected patients are young, often in their twenties and thirties, often the same age as their caregivers, and so it is perhaps natural that they turn to them for comfort and understanding. This is particularly true if the caregiver and the patient share common orientations. As Jason R. commented:

> Sometimes, because I'm gay also, if they are gay, there's some camaraderie. They feel they can trust you, I think. Sometimes with drug users, there's a particularly strong feeling that they need to feel some companionship with you. They get friendly, they need a lot of people to talk to. They have a hard time, and maybe they can't tell everything to the people in their lives, so they just like to talk to you [the nurse] about things.

Another nurse who practiced in-home care said of her patients: "You're supposed to be the mother they never had, the sister they never had. You're supposed to know all about the disease and how to deal with it. Most patients feel that they can keep loading onto you, and you're going to be able to cope with all of it."

The most common emotions that the patient experiences and that the nurse must in some way respond to are sorrow and anger. There is sorrow because HIV disease is ultimately a terminal diagnosis. Death may be delayed and treatments developed in the last decade do put off death for some time, but ultimately HIV disease is fatal. This is the message that the diagnosis brings, and it is a message that the nurse has to contend with while striving to care for the patient. As George T. said:

> So you come toddling in as the nurse, all efficient, doing your thing, meaning absolutely nothing negative, you just want to get your job done so you can get your chart in and run out the door because you've got so much to do, and here's this person who has just been told that it's HIV, and to them it means death. They need a lot, even those who don't say it.

Some patients are more expressive than others and some groups seem more able than others to set up systems for coping. Nora M., whose patients were poor, mostly IVDUs, had this to say:

> The drug users are not able to advocate for themselves in the same way as gay patients. They are very, very, fearful, and they are not able to express their fears. You find that you have to advocate for them. It's very hard to reach them; it's hard to get their confidence or their trust. With gays, it's much easier. With the drug users, it's much more difficult to get them to verbalize what's really going on, because most of them have never explored what's happening. Most of them have just come off drugs and suddenly they're in treatment programs. They don't really know where they're at or where they've come from. It is usually anger; anger is the thing you have to deal with.

> Anger and fear, and fear is usually unexpressed, from my experience. They can't say, "I'm afraid," but you can see it in their faces. They know what's going on. They know they have a terminal disease. They may not tell you as fast as other groups, but they know, they know.

Fear may be unexpressed but anger is commonly encountered. Two nurses said that the reason they had left direct, hands-on nursing of HIV-infected patients was because they had had to face so much anger. Because the nurse sees the patient often, she or he often feels the brunt of the patient's distress. As one nurse, who moved from direct care to an administrative position, said of a home-care patient.

> One woman was real sad. She had been an IV drug user back in the early 1980s, and she had cleaned up her act, and she was diagnosed with HIV in 1987, five years later. I've never seen such rage in all my life. This woman was so angry, and everybody could understand the anger, but we had to take turns seeing her because we would go in to see her, and she would just start yelling at us. The first thing she did was to start shooting questions at us to find out how much we knew about HIV. She was trying to see what we knew. Then she would go into these tirades. She had been mistreated in hospitals. They misdiagnosed one of her infections. She had side effects from the medication that could have been avoided. She was one of these medical disasters. It really belongs on "60 Minutes." It all went wrong and it went wrong in the wrong person. So she was just impossible. To deal with the situation, the supervisor would have us take turns because nobody could deal with her rage.

Patients are frequently angry. Dealing with this anger can exhaust nurses. In addition, nurses may find that their patients anger them. Some patients are cooperative and compliant. Some are a pleasure to care for. Some are not. They can make providing care very difficult. As the nurse quoted above went on to say:

> Sometimes no matter what I do, it's wrong, and I ask, "Why am I wasting my time with this person?" I hear constantly from nurses how frustrating it is and how sometimes you just want to shake somebody. On the one hand, you have patients who are taking your advice and eating properly and taking their pills and everything, and then you've got this other person who's not listening to a word you're saying. He's constantly complaining about his symptoms. When you tell him to take his pills, he won't. You feel kind of nasty, and like

> saying, "Well, don't tell me about your symptoms, if you're not going to do a thing I say." It's like, "Why are you wasting my time?"

Patients who do not comply are a source of great tension to nurses. Patients who reject some or all of what nurses offer break the relation of mutuality that underlies nursing. Because HIV disease is bringing large numbers of patients into the medical system who have difficulty following rules and directions, many nurses, unfamiliar with the populations most afflicted with HIV disease, are being challenged to revise their expectations of the nursing experience.

Jean C. described how, when a patient rejected her care, she shifted her attention from the patient to the patient's mother:

> My first AIDS patient was a prisoner who came home from the hospital after treatment and I was his home-care nurse. He lived in a very horrible place, and his mother was having a lot of difficulty trying to handle him. He was very, very angry. I don't think I ever got through to him. He died angry. It was a fight for me to care for him. He didn't want me to come. He was very sick, of course, and eventually he let me clean him up because it was just so uncomfortable. But he slept on a couch. He wouldn't let me get him a hospital bed. He got to the point where he couldn't walk. I had to do everything for him. But he never opened up, and the only satisfaction I got from that was I helped his mother in dealing with it all. She did her very best, under the circumstances. She was very good; she was not a very smart woman, but she worked every day and she had lots of children, lots of problems. Yet she took the best care she could of her son. I think that's where I got satisfaction out of that situation, that I could be a help to her.

HIV-infected patients who are gay, IVDUs, blacks or females do not in any way conform to what Erving Goffman has described as the ideal person in American society: "a young, married, white, urban, northern, heterosexual Protestant father of college education, fully employed, of good complexion, weight and height and a recent record in sports" (quoted in Perin 1988: 145). HIV-infected patients are imperfect people according to the norms of American society, and encountering them, or, in the case of nurses, having to care for them in large numbers, can result in a kind of culture shock for those who are unprepared. These patients can be threatening. Indeed, they are threatening on an elementary physical level. They are contagious.

Although HIV disease is rather hard to contract—it does not seem to be transmitted through respiration, for example—it can and has been transmitted through needle punctures, a common occupational hazard for nurses. The first nurse to contract HIV disease through work died in 1992. Yet the nurses I interviewed did not seem overly concerned about acquiring HIV disease from patient contact. Only four nurses I interviewed said they were apprehensive about catching HIV disease. Most had come to terms in different ways with the risk their patients posed. Marcia B., who was working in an emergency room at the beginning of the epidemic, said:

> There are still people who will tell you, "Well, you never know." I had a physician at a meeting say recently, "Well, you don't know what they are not telling us about this virus," and to hear something like that amazes me. You talk about being scared. I should be very nervous, because with those first few patients, we took no precautions. We were touching body fluids constantly, blood got all over our hands.

But all the nurses I interviewed said they were very careful now. As one noted: "We follow universal precautions. I just got tested. I get tested every year." They do not discount the danger, but they do believe that HIV disease is primarily transmitted through sexual contact or contamination with infected blood. As Carey M. said: "I guess I've worked it out. I've been a nurse for almost twenty years, and I wonder about all the needle sticks I had that I didn't worry about before. I couldn't work here if I didn't really believe that the way the disease is transmitted is the way they're telling us."

These nurses rely on time-tested methods of infection control: cleanliness and limited contact. Some do, however, develop a feeling of fatalism. One nurse said: "I think my friends think I should be more worried. I was bitten by an AIDS patient back in 1987, and I've had a few needle sticks. But for some reason I guess I'm not that worried. If it's meant to be, I believe that if I'm meant to get it, so be it."

Other nurses find that dealing with the possibility of infection is an issue that doesn't die. It is not settled once and for all; it recurs and has to be worked through each time. As Chris T. explained:

> Before I took this job, I think I was actually lucky, because before I took the job I thought about all of these issues, and I sort of accepted the risks as a part of the job, and I worked it out ahead of time. My family had some reaction to it, not tremendous really. My uncle asked me if I made sure to wash my hands a lot. I didn't have a lot of real negative stuff that a lot of people do have. What I did when I took this job, I said to myself, "Okay, it's spread like hepatitis, I

> believe the epidemiology." A lot of people didn't buy it at the time and they still don't buy it. But I did, and ergo, if I follow the precautions, the blood and body fluid precautions for hepatitis, then I will be safe. But then I was stuck with a needle. I stuck myself actually. It wasn't an avoidable accident. I stuck myself through a pair of gloves, and my bubble burst. They didn't even have a test for HIV then. It was 1984. I was upset for a while, and then the test came out, and I took it, and I tested negative. I was really rational and empirical about it. Nobody had come down with AIDS from caring for patients yet. I kind of looked at that and tried not to think about it too terribly much because I had chosen this work. And, you know, hepatitis is a risk and it's a much greater risk than HIV. The fact that there is a risk is not new. Nurses went in and took care of polio patients, dengue fever, cholera, etc. It [HIV disease] seems very overwhelming now because I think we've had a long period when we felt comfortable. People expected different things from their work and one of the things people expected was that they would be safe. You have to think all these things through, and it's a real process. It's not a process that ever goes away. I think what happens is that an accident happens, you get upset, but you deal with it; you think about it, you learn some more and get some more information, you talk to people, you work it through and you feel better. And if something else happens, you may get some sort of a reaction but it's not as severe as the first time. It's sort of cyclical but it's on an upward spiral.

Many of the nurses in this study continue "to work it through" because HIV disease is not an easy disease to get used to. Fear of contagion is real. Keeping the fear under control takes a number of forms. Concentrating on the comparative risks of contracting HIV disease and hepatitis is one way. Focusing on the efficacy of using gloves is another. Just trying not to think about it is another. Each nurse seems to construct her or his own method of acknowledging the danger while putting it into perspective. If this wasn't possible, these nurses could not do their jobs.

For nurses who remembered when serious, life-threatening, infectious disease was a fact of life, the adjustment was relatively easy. Several nurses I interviewed trained in the 1950s and early 1960s and they recalled an era before antibiotics. Alice D. commented:

> Nurses have always had these fears, but historically it has been so much a part of life. Up until the late 1950s and early 1960s, communicable diseases were so much a part of life, and so much a part of

> nursing, that you just didn't go into nursing unless you were willing to take care of patients with contagious diseases.

As Carey M. said:

> I'm old enough to remember polio, and I'm old enough to remember all this other stuff that happened. When I went into nursing there was still a communicable disease hospital in lower Manhattan. I remember Willard Parker hospital where the polio patients were. But younger nurses probably don't understand that. I think that a lot of people who went into nursing and maybe medicine, too, in the sixties didn't bargain for this.

Before childhood diseases were conquered, people's expectations and life experiences were quite different from today. As one commentator has said about life before antibiotics:

> How ordinary it was for someone to miss a year of school while recovering from a debilitating disease, to postpone a marriage while nursing a relative, to spend some time in a sanatorium. Ear infections, common in childhood, could deafen people for life. Strep throat led to rheumatic fever whose victims died young. (Smith 1990: 389)

Now most people expect to be healthy most of their lives.

The advent of antibiotics and their widespread use in the past thirty years created the healthiest generation in history. The younger nurses in this study grew up experiencing health as a constant and illness as an aberration. HIV disease has demonstrated how unusual this was. It has underscored the vulnerability of the human body and the number of pathogens anxious to colonize it. This is a lesson in humility. As Roberta M. said:

> I think most of them in obstetrics have learned to protect themselves and I think some of the surgeons have gotten out of medicine. Yet it's a very real honest-to-God fear, when you think especially of places like emergency rooms where people are standing in blood. Five, six, ten years ago we didn't pay attention to blood. Washing it off our hands, that was all. Now I use gloves all the time. I'm absolutely changed. I'm not so cavalier. I've just become a lot more respectful of the virus.

Alice D. called HIV disease

> a whole different ball game. There's no getting away from it. People used to think, "Well, I'll work in obstetrics [to escape HIV disease]," but now that's the worst of all in terms of blood exposure. So it's across the spectrum now. There's no hiding. I think we have to face it head on, and we have to educate health care workers for the realities of practice, and we have to support each other. And we must not criticize nurses who do have fears. It's not an unreasonable fear.

Many of the nurses I interviewed said that they actually felt safer taking care of HIV-infected patients who were identified as such, because when they dealt with such patients, they were always protective of themselves. As Lore H. said: "It's the people you don't know the HIV results of that you should be more worried about. You should take the same precautions with every patient, but you may not." Nina H. agreed. She described delaying telling her mother she was working with HIV-infected patients:

> I didn't tell her for quite a few months that I was working with HIV patients because I knew what I'd get and it wasn't going to be support. When I finally told her, I got exactly what I thought I was going to get, full of fear. But what I said to her was, "I know who I'm working with." When you're on the floor, and I've experienced this myself, you're just too busy. You say to yourself, "This person has breast cancer," and in your head you think, "She's not HIV." So you don't slip on the gloves when you're taking blood, and yet you don't know. You just don't know. So here I think there's safety in knowing the patients are HIV-infected. There's safety in knowing who you are dealing with and you take precautions.

Precautions include being careful about mixing and administering drugs, many of which are highly toxic. Many nurses said that the toxicity of the drugs for HIV disease was a concern. The drugs are very potent. One nurse feared that they were sometimes doing more harm than good. Also, both nurse and patient can be at risk when the drug is administered. When giving aerosol pentamidine treatments, for example, the chances that the nurse will inhale some of the drug are high, unless an enclosed, airtight booth, costing about $35,000, is used. Most clinics do not have such booths.

A much more immediate concern for the nurses in the study was the possibility of contracting TB from their patients. One nurse told me that several of the nurses on her unit had contracted TB in the past year. They did not simply become seropositive, as many nurses do, but they actually developed the active disease. One nurse in this study also developed active TB, which was a complete surprise because she had no symptoms. Only a routine skin test, followed by an X-ray, revealed a lesion on her lung. Another nurse mentioned that pneumonia had been common among her staff during the past year. The resurgence of these diseases, particularly in drug-resistant forms, is very disturbing. As Lena F. said:

> I don't know what's coming down the pike. But I think that what's going to happen with many of these opportunistic infections is that, because we're hitting them with the most potent chemicals we can possibly hit them with now, the germ will eventually become immune to whatever we're hitting it with. That's what the history of antibiotic therapy tells us. When that immunity develops, then you have to go the next step up. But with these [infections], we're using our big guns now. What do we use when the big guns fail? I don't know.

Alice D. commented:

> We have seen more seroconversion for TB and I think in a way that may present a greater occupational health hazard than AIDS, because what distinguishes AIDS from all previous communicable disease is that, on the bad side, it's not curable if you get it and there's no vaccine. But the good side is that it's not very easy to catch, whereas TB is much easier. I think from an overall public health point of view, TB presents a more serious threat even though most TB is curable and people aren't so afraid of it. But we're seeing more and more TB in AIDS patients, especially in drug abusers, and we've gotten a little lax about isolation precautions and all that. We don't take it quite as seriously now because there's a pill for it. But it's a real threat.

The many manifestations and ramifications of HIV disease challenge nurses' and patients' expectations about the course of illness and the expectation of cure. The disease also challenges expectations about personal integrity and autonomy, especially because so many HIV-infected patients now exhibit signs of dementia. HIV-infected patients can be kept alive quite a long time, but the benefits of longevity are sometimes outweighed by brain infection and the lesions that produce dementia. In their second interviews, many nurses in this study said that the major change they had noticed since I last spoke with them was that now most of their patients eventually became demented. This is hard for nurses, for patients, and for families. As Bob G. said: "You don't expect people your own age to be demented."

Dementia complicates care in many ways. As outpatients, demented patients do not come for appointments, nor do they follow drug regimens. When they are in the hospital, they present many management problems. Because the patients do not realize how frail they are, nurses have to restrain them. They try to get out of bed themselves, frequently falling and risking fractures.

Demented patients can lose their personalities. This is not only distressing to their caregivers, it can also mean that care has to be premised on a new set of expectations. As Toby B. said about one of her patients:

> We had a team conference this morning on one of the patients. He came in just to get some IV medication for an infection, and then he was supposed to go home, but he had a seizure. So they were working him up for a seizure, they had him all set, and he had another seizure. Now he's totally organic. He has lesions all over his brain. From being a very quiet, demure person, he has completely revised his personality. He's very demanding, pulling out things, he's pulling out his IVs, he's frightened. When he does come into reality, all he says is, "I'm scared." We can't spend the whole day holding his hand, so we've tried to get his family and friends to come in during the day, and then at night we sedate him enough so at least he'll get some rest.

HIV disease turns many of our expectations upside down. It is a threat to the old order because it strikes at the heart of the biomedical world view dominant in medicine for the past generation. Although the manifestations of HIV disease are becoming better known, it still remains an elusive quarry. The medical magic bullets so effective in the last twenty-five years are only partially effective against this disease. They only work against its symptoms.

The theories on which American medicine is founded do not satisfactorily explain HIV disease. The germ theory of disease supports the notion that the HIV virus causes the disease, but so far the research predicated on this theory has borne little fruit. What this does is remove one of the supports nurses have relied on in the past thirty years: the conviction that the disease or condition is a known quantity and that there is a remedy or a treatment specific to it. HIV disease removes this certainty.

Thus HIV disease makes unusual demands on nurses' and other health care workers' intellectual powers. That which they thought was settled proves to be unsettled. That which they thought was true may not be true after all. What is known is only partial, not anywhere near complete. This produces unease, and in Freud's words, "unpleasure": "The source of this unpleasure is the demand made upon the mind by anything that is new, the psychical expenditure that it requires, the uncertainty, mounting up to anxious expectancy that it brings with it" (quoted in Perin 1988: 172).

HIV disease threatens nurses' intellectual certainties, but *HIV-infected patients* threaten nurses' moral equilibrium as well, because they call into question the meanings by which we in America live. "Every anomaly or 'stranger' announce [*sic*] that they cannot be accounted for by concepts that organize a familiar field of meaning" (Perin 1988: 146). HIV-infected patients pose a challenge to the categories we live by, categories that determine who is worthy and who is not. More often than not in New York City, HIV-infected patients are the "failures" of society. Many HIV-infected patients are not "worthy," by American standards, and yet they require care. In caring for them, many nurses fear they too may be included in the category of those without value (Gee 1989).

Like peoples in other cultures, "Americans attribute dangerous social powers to whatever and whomever are seen as being marginal to or in transition between clearly defined social statuses" (Perin 1988: 10). Thus HIV-infected patients are frequently seen as polluting and less than human. Because AIDS patients upset the usual order, they are subject to rejection, a rejection that is based on, and which seeks to maintain, old practices and beliefs.

Most HIV-infected patients in New York City are different from their caregivers and present challenges to their caregivers' established ways of thinking and doing. But rather than turning away from HIV-infected patients because they present so many differences, the nurses in this study have chosen another way to cope with the dissonance these patients produce. They turn toward rather than away from their patients. And in turning toward them, they have found a way to move beyond the stigmas of race, homosexuality, and drug use. They rely on the concept of "patient" that includes, rather than excludes, these groups. They do this by focusing on what joins them to others, their humanity, and by ignoring that which separates them, their social status.

The nurses in this study have overcome the fears and distrust that a new and uncontrollable disease naturally inspires. This has been achieved through a conscious and determined effort to see patients with HIV disease as, first and foremost, people in need, and only secondarily as gays, IVDUs, and minorities. They have done this by developing a capacity similar to Keats's "negative capability—the capability of so negating their identity as to be imaginatively open to the complex and never very certain reality around them" (Crapanzano 1985: xxii). In so doing, they are able to see their patients as human beings like themselves. They do not fear them and do not seek to exclude them from the circle of those who deserve care.

Chapter 5
Holism and Connection: Providing Care

The essence of the kind of nursing the nurses in this study practice is "to be there for their patients." Simons describes this as "attention [that] includes more than mere physical presence. It reflects a being 'in tune' with each other, an awareness of unique personhood" (quoted in Benner 1989: 13).

Being there for people means being open and accessible, ready to listen, to recommend, to make referrals, to see that things get done, to do things oneself. It is the stance toward patients that the nurses I interviewed described when they talked about taking a holistic view of the patient. It means considering all aspects of the patient's situation, including medical issues, family status, psychological functioning, ethnicity, sexual preference, and the like. It can also mean getting the mop oneself to clean up a spill rather than waiting for the aide to do it.

HIV-infected patients in New York City are particularly in need of comprehensive care because so many of them lack family supports. Gay men and IVDUs frequently live alone, and, as they become more debilitated, they become dependent on formal services both for ordinary domestic requirements and for medical and nursing care. HIV-infected women are often the single caretakers of families. They and those dependent on them need help with cooking, shopping, and paying bills, all those tasks that healthy people perform for themselves, or which could be managed for them by other family members. The isolation of many HIV-infected patients means that they need many and diverse services in order to live with their disease. Thus the desire of the nurses in this study to consider the whole person in their nursing practice meshes with the needs of HIV-infected patients.

This readiness to commit oneself and one's resources on behalf of another is the first step in forging a connection with patients. And a personal connection with the patient is necessary if the nurse is to see the patient as a three-dimensional person. For nearly all of the nurses I interviewed, establishing a personal connection with patients was extremely important. Through this personal commitment, these nurses approach their patients as people like themselves—a critical beginning if they are to transcend the social divisions that typically place gays, IVDUs, blacks, and other minorities at the margins of American society. Once established, the personal connection between nurse and patient is the mechanism through which differences of class, race, and gender can be negotiated.

It is through knowing the patient as an individual that these nurses individualize care, tailor it to the particular patient, and take into account the intangibles that affect illness and recovery. When these nurses reflected on their roles, particularly on how their roles differ from those of doctors, it is this aspect they emphasized. As Sally G., who was the primary caregiver in an HIV unit, said:

> When I describe what a nurse practitioner is, everybody always says, "Oh, that's just like a doctor." I guess the thing I would like people to see is that what I do as a nurse practitioner, a lot of the things I do, do cross over into medicine; it's a really autonomous role, and you do take care of things that doctors usually do, but there are parts of that that I really believe I do better, because I think I'm much more ready to really listen to how events or diagnoses or treatments are affecting the patient. I also think I really spend a lot of time making somebody understand the medicines or how to treat their pain or what a diagnosis means. I feel that, when I'm with a patient, my patient feels that I care about their status, and that I understand what they're supposed to do about it. I feel that my chances that this is all going to happen are better than a lot of physicians', because I think even a lot of physicians who try to do things like this can't do it as well, because they are just so far removed they don't understand why a patient doesn't understand, or what it is about what they say that patients just don't understand or can't comply with. What I do is assess how people are affected by their illness or affected by their diagnosis or affected by things in their lives that are making them have physical complaints. I think that I assess these better than a physician. I think it's always been nursing's strong emphasis, that's why I'm tuned into it, to be more holistic, to understand social aspects of illness and health.

HIV disease has been called nursing's disease because most of the patient's needs are those requiring nursing knowledge—for example, comfort care, pain control, nutrition, and elimination. As Alice D. commented:

> Their [HIV-infected patients'] health problems really fall into the nurse's domain. There is so little that medicine can do, and there is no cure. There are some cures for opportunistic infections, but basically what they need is good nursing care, good supportive care, both physical and psychological, and spiritual and emotional [care]. I think it's really an area in which nurses can have a great impact, because a lot of what's needed is keeping patients free of pain, or trying to keep their weight on, keep them from becoming malnourished. They come in with massive diarrhea and we try to get that under control, keep their skin clean and dry, keep the skin from breaking down. We help them with their self-care deficits. So many of them are so tired, they can't bathe themselves, they can't shampoo their hair, all the little things that need doing. They also need emotional help. Many of them feel a great deal of guilt. There are many who feel they can't share this with their families. That's where nursing can do a great deal of good.

The care needed by HIV-infected patients has to take into account all sorts of problems that might not otherwise be considered clinical, from wills to custody to homelessness. One nurse in a municipal hospital, whose patients were mostly street people, said she tried to teach her patients how to keep clean and decently fed. She saw herself as a one-person referral bureau to services for the homeless in New York City.

These nurses try to see the whole picture: they are interested in how the various aspects of their patients' lives come together and affect their illness and their care. This focus on connection is central to how the nurses I spoke with view their role. They believe that a patient's experience of illness depends on the interaction of a host of factors that might appear on the surface to have nothing to do with disease. This is why, according to Emma J., nurses are in a position to make a significant contribution to how patient care for persons with AIDS is organized:

> Nurses have always considered themselves holistic health providers who are interested in how a disease affects the person's entire life, not just whether they need lab work done, or if they need to change medicines or whatever, and there's so much room for that in AIDS, to help people deal with multiple issues like control or body image or plans or lovers or family, etc. I think some of the things that are important in AIDS are things that nurses really do well.

It is not always the big things that make life miserable. It can be the conditions which, in another patient, would be considered minor. But in an HIV-infected patient these conditions can become major. Diarrhea is one such condition. HIV-disease diarrhea can be extremely hard to control. As Gladys R. said:

> When we first started out [in the AIDS unit], we had a lot of PCP, then we had KS, then we had TB, then everybody had toxoplasmosis, and then cryptomeningitis. We had a lot of crypto [-sporidium, a gastrointestinal protozoa]. My God, if you don't really love what you're doing, you don't come back once you've met that, because the smell of the stool—crypto produces constant diarrhea, and that smell, you can smell it far away from their door. I remember one guy, I cleaned him three times in the one attempt. I cleaned him and fixed him up, then more diarrhea. I took him out of bed and I had to put him right back. You know that's so devastating to them. It is so devastating for them, and for you too, because the thing is that you have nothing to offer them. That's really sometimes the hardest part of the job. You haven't anything to offer, in the sense of being medically able to help them very much.

It is at this point that nurses begin to rely on a different set of skills. When clinical treatments have achieved all they can, what is left is human compassion and empathy. As Emily D. explained:

> I've had nurses say to me, "I feel like I'm not doing anything. I feel so useless, so helpless." For example, when I have somebody with chronic diarrhea and we have tried every medicine under the sun, and nothing has worked, and the patient still has cramping pain, it's very hard. So sometimes I have to say to them, "I wish we could do something but we can't; maybe if you avoid certain foods, it will make your life a little easier, but I can't make it all pleasant again." I've found with my patients, in this kind of situation, when I said that to them, sometimes I would get anger, but usually I wouldn't. Usually, I would get a certain resignation.

Emily went on to say:

> When you let people know that you really can't control an aspect [of their disease], and that everything has been tried, but nothing really works, then sometimes, as long as they can complain to you about it, it makes them feel better. I had this one patient. He was always nauseous. We had tried everything; we couldn't do anything about his nausea. He would say to me, "I just need to complain about being nauseous today, just let me complain a little bit. I know you can't do anything." So I would sit there and go "Hum-um," and that's all he

> wanted. Because the other issue too is, particularly for the patients who are well connected to other people, they realize their friends have a limited tolerance for listening to all the gory details. As one of my patients said to me, "You know, if I can complain to you about how I feel, then when my friends come over, I can be sociable with them." And I would tell him, "That's one of the reasons I'm here."

There is a double vision at the center of this kind of nursing. These nurses balance two views of the patient at once. They are intent on doing all the monitoring, performing all the procedures, bringing the medication, and documenting the patient's condition. At the same time, they are alert to social and psychological factors that will bear on the outcome of treatment. They are "concerned" about their patients and alert to the messages their patients send (Benner 1989).

Thus, the perspective from which these nurses view their patients and from which they draw their inspiration encourages them to look at the needs of their patients and to use these needs as the basis for planning, instead of relying on institutional rules and regulations. Such an inclusive view of the patient as a whole person leads nurses like the ones in this study to consider and deal with issues of patient care that other health professionals, because of their narrower focus, can ignore. The nurses in this study do not feel comfortable with a narrow definition of their role. Even physicians who are caring and conscientious will draw lines where these nurses would not. As Gretchen S., who practices in a municipal hospital, said:

> There are some doctors who go out of their way to help; there's one doctor here who's really gone out of his way to fill out the compassionate care forms [for experimental drugs]. There's a lot of paperwork in order to get these drugs. They're only given on an individualized basis, so you have to see if the patient will fit into the category, and this doc has really tried to do that. He's very meticulous, and he's gone out of his way to get different lab values to make sure that it's all complete for someone when they come to clinic. But when I mentioned that there was a lawyer who was available, who was willing to come to clinic twice a month to deal with custody cases, he didn't want to know from custody cases. He didn't want to know; it wasn't his role. And I feel very strongly about the custody cases especially. If someone has kids, what happens to the kids after they die is very important. When you address this issue with people, you don't say *when you die*. You say *if something happens to you*. But, otherwise, these kids get knocked around in the foster care system. It's pretty awful, and people need to know that is a potential problem. There are all these

> fathers who suddenly resurrect out of nowhere. Or one's mother says she will take them, but they never sign papers and maybe the kids go into foster care for two or three months until it gets settled. But there are ways to address it. And I think it's very important. But this doc didn't want to address it. He didn't want to talk about it.

This nurse and many of the others I interviewed made it part of their practice to raise these issues with patients. Gretchen went on to say: "I try to do the topics they seem to want more, like child custody and wills. Just because people are poor doesn't mean they don't have something they want to pass on to someone else."

A holistic concept of nursing is a necessary part of physical care also, because HIV disease involves so many different bodily systems. In order to provide proper care, a nurse has to be attentive to how the disease might affect parts of the body beyond the immediate site of an infection. She has to keep in mind the totality of the patient's body. As Stephanie C., who had more than seven years of experience in HIV care, remarked:

> The disease changes. We're constantly finding new aspects of the HIV infection. I'll just give you one example. The candida esophagitis [a yeast infection] that goes down the esophagus, we're discovering that sometimes it's not what we thought it was. There are new studies which show that it could be direct HIV infection of the esophagus as well as herpes and CMV [cytomegalovirus]. It could be one or a combination of the above. We saw PCP [pneumocystis carinii pneumonia] in bone marrow the other day, in a woman who recently died. It is going places we had never seen. Nobody had seen a case of it in the bone marrow before. We already look for MAI [mycobacterium avium-intracellulare] in the bone marrow and now we'll have to look for PCP.

The comprehensive concept of nursing that these nurses practice is expressed first in their attentiveness to the patient's physical condition. HIV-infected patients can be very unstable. Their condition can change rapidly. One nurse in home care, who said he was never sure what condition his patients would be in when he went to see them, called HIV disease "a real roller coaster." He described one case:

> During the summer, there was a gentleman I would go to see every morning. I had this routine of going first thing in the morning because he lived close to me, and it made life easier. It was finished early in the day for him and for me and we were both happy. It was a

> Friday morning, it was raining out, and I went to his apartment and knocked on the door, and there was no answer. And, of course, if there is no answer, you panic. So finally someone answered and it was the man's lover-roommate. He had been asleep, and he told me that my patient had bled to death the night before. I almost freaked out. You're with death all the time, and when it takes a long time, it's not a shock, but when it's that fast, it makes no sense to you. It can be really tough when you're out there on your own.

Another nurse in hospital nursing agreed:

> Certainly their disease is very unique. You learn something new about it every day, and you can see things that you don't see in anything else. You see patients who develop confusion very quickly. You'll see them fully alert and oriented at 9 A.M., and at noon they're gone. Patients can go from being very stable to being very critical, like in three hours. You see patients who have CMV retinitis [cytomegalovirus infection] who see very well when they come in here, and they're blind when they leave. You see people who come in here with what might be a simple case of pneumonia—it may not be PCP, it may be another kind of pneumonia—and they end up on ventilators.

HIV disease's unpredictability, coupled with its complexity, means that more than the usual attentiveness is required. As Ethel R. commented:

> For example, the doctor orders this medication, and you give it to the patient. Then you walk in later and you see the man beet red. It's an allergic reaction. It's up to you, the nurse; you have to stop the medication, you have to page the doctor to come in and order the medication to counter the allergy and the reaction, and you have to go all over again with something else. Sometimes the patient will say, "I don't want it; it's going to make me sick like the other one." So you have to teach them. "No, this is a different one. You do have this infection. We have to try different medications. Yes, you are sensitive to that medicine, but that doesn't mean you're sensitive to this."

One nurse compared HIV nursing to general nursing thus:

> You're using your basic medical surgical skills and background; you use med-surg in everything, but then there are various signs of OIs [opportunistic infections] which you need to pick up on. With a lot of the medication, you have to watch their renal values, you have to

> watch their glucose values, their pancreatic values. The medications carry more side effects, too. You have to be alert to the hydration and to a patient's nutritional status, and how far into the illness they are because there are various factors that stop working in the nutritional area as they get further into HIV. They can't eat and they develop a wasting syndrome.

Patients will often have several conditions at the same time, each a major problem. They might have pneumonia and TB and syphilis along with less serious infections such as thrush or psoriasis. Complicated drug regimens for each disease have to be instituted, followed by close monitoring.

Thus, in order to care for HIV patients, nurses need first-rate clinical skills and a continuing interest in learning. They have to be alert and knowledgeable. Many nurses said that one of their satisfactions came from meeting the demands of clinical care. It's a pleasure, they said, to have the knowledge and to be able to use it. Not every nurse has the requisite skills. An administrator at one hospital told me that she had had several nurses who wanted to work in the AIDS unit but who just weren't good enough to do it. It is complex work. Lore H., who was attracted by the complexity of the disease, said:

> There are so many different systems that can be affected in any individual, and so you might have to couple respiratory therapy with cancer and with this and with that. It's so many multiple systems that can be affected. You're dealing with them all. You have to balance them all, while thinking about what works best for the patient all the time.

As part of this effort to work out what's best for the patient, these nurses frequently look ahead to what the next level of care should be. This is what Benner (1984) describes as "forward thinking." They anticipate and initiate. Gretchen S. noticed at her hospital that more women were appearing with HIV disease, and so she instituted regular pelvic exams for her clinic patients over the objections of many on the HIV-clinic staff; they wanted to send the patients to the regular Ob-Gyn clinic. But Gretchen said: "The physician assistants thought I was crazy when I tried to do the pelvics. I got a real sense that people really thought I was crazy. People said, 'Why would you want to do that for? Why bother? It's yucky. Are you crazy? Just send them downstairs.'"

But according to her code, this nurse would have been remiss if she hadn't done pelvic exams, since infection in women often manifests itself in the reproductive organs. Another nurse said that the infectious disease doctor in her hospital didn't even order a gynecological exam for a female patient who came in with a fever until the nurse suggested it. In insisting on the gynecological exam, this nurse is certainly doing for the patient what the patient cannot do for herself, but what she would do if she had the nurse's knowledge.

Along with attention to the patient's physical condition, these nurses strive to keep the patient in touch with life and with normality. Most nurses saw sustaining the patient's hope as part of their job. This can be as simple as a bath and a short trip outside the room. For both patient and nurse it can be a pleasurable experience. This is how Gladys R. described what she enjoyed about nursing:

> I love bedside nursing. Yes, I do. I like to be able to see my patient get well and go home, or my patient is sick and needs my help. I'm there to give the help he needs, to help that patient get over that hump, and I'll look at him and he might say, "Thank you, I'm feeling much better today. Yes, my breathing is better." And I say, "Okay," and I brush their hair, or comb their hair, and clean them up nicely, and sit them up, and say, "Okay, I'm going to take you out of bed for half an hour." I take them down to the patient's lounge in a wheelchair, and let them sit there, even for five minutes, and then bring them back. It gives me great satisfaction to know I did this, and that it helps the patient. At least they had a little bit of life again.

With this sort of activity, these nurses keep their patients within the circle of social value. They strive to maintain their patients' social place and meaning. They do not limit their interaction to a formal exchange of information. Lena F. described clinic days as "fun"; Gretchen S. said:

> I don't have that much time with them. It's not like I have a whole hour to talk to people, but people know that I am there in some way. Clinic is really crazy. Sometimes I'm really ditzy, because I'm always forgetting something, and I tell the patients to remind me. "If you want a chest X-ray, remind me." "If you need Motrin, remind me again." It's really a chaotic scene. It's not really a scene which is conducive to any kind of real thoughtful processes, because while I'm doing all this, I'm trying to maintain the energy for people, because I have a lot of energy myself. I try to let people know that they're special. When I come through the waiting room, there are some that I know, and they address me, and I address them. "You look great today!" or "It's a great shirt you're wearing." That's not unnoticed, that I don't just walk in and pick up the chart. And I've gotten stuff back because of that. Someone last week said, "Thank

you, just thanks for being there for all of us." And he wasn't even my patient.

Stephanie C. arranged for a patient to display his photographs in the hospital. She wanted him to feel that he was still a productive and contributing member of society. She said:

> I have a patient who is a very talented photographer, very artistic, and very bored. He's going to be in the hospital for three weeks; he has toxo [toxoplasmosis] and he is going to get medication. And we're going to work him for other things too, like possible CMV retinitis. But he has photographs of Liz Taylor and Tina Turner. He's had exclusive sessions with them. He's really very talented, and so, right now, we're planning a show for him in the hospital. It's important to him. The message he gives me is that he wants to keep active, professionally and personally.

The nurses I spoke with encourage their patients to maintain a normal life as long as they can. But with HIV disease there inevitably comes a time when preparing for death becomes necessary. Paula T. described herself as becoming "the death nurse in her hospital," and another nurse remarked, rather ruefully, that she seemed to have a talent for death.

A good death is the last gift the nurse can give the patient. Keeping patients company while they die is a last act of connection and the ultimate recognition that those suffering are valued. It can be the most intimate experience of all, and it can be as important for the nurse as for the patient. Carol H., who had little experience of death before she became an HIV nurse, said of the first HIV-infected patient she cared for who died:

> I remember the first one who died who I was very close to. I think what made him special was that he was so at peace with himself. When he died, it was okay, and death then was very new to me. I was rather unusual in that most people who come into AIDS work usually have some experience [with death], but I didn't. I knew no one who had AIDS, so it was all new. And you're really sharing; it's really intimate. They let us in. They let us in so readily, and that's really extraordinary. As I sat with him as he was dying, it reminded me of sitting with women in labor, giving birth. It's a very intimate experience. You don't know when it's going to happen, and you have to have the patience to wait for it. And it's momentous. It's happening and you have to give yourself to it.

Several nurses said that some patients wait for permission to die or wait for their favorite nurse to be on duty before they die. Toby B., who nurses in a voluntary hospital, said that the staff and most of the patients on her unit were very honest about death; this enabled them to work toward "good deaths." As she said: "We got into helping people be comfortable about letting go and talking about it and letting them know that it was okay. I don't believe in mercy killing, so you can't do that, but you can certainly give someone permission to let go."

She went on to describe one patient

> who was at the end, but his parents kept coming in and saying, "Hang in there, don't go, there's a cure around the corner," at the same time that his [the patient's] lover was accepting his death. The parents came in during the day and the lover in the evening. Finally, I told the lover to go get a cup of coffee and I went into the patient's room, and I said to him, "It's okay, you can go." He was breathing slowly, only a few times per minute, and lo and behold, he just stopped, like that. I was flabbergasted. He did what I told him.

Many nurses recognized that their role continued beyond death. They became the link between the patient's past, his present, and his future. Like Dr. Rieux in Albert Camus' *The Plague*, they saw themselves as among those who "should bear witness in favor of those plague-stricken people; so that some memorial of the injustice and outrage done them might endure; and to state quite simply what we learn in time of pestilence: that there are more things to admire in men than to despise" (1948: 178).

The nurse who arranged for her patient to show his photographs also proposed a program whereby patients themselves might create a record their families could retain. The program would have enabled patients to produce their own videotapes so that their families, their children particularly, could have kept an image of what they were like before they became terminally ill. She said:

> One young mother looked me in the face, she was holding a two-year-old by the hand, and she said, "He won't know who I am. I'll be dead and he won't remember me. He won't know what I look like; he won't know where I came from." And I had an epiphany, you know, like James Joyce, and I had this picture of this whole thing, that if we could capture these women doing a sort of family review, or whatever it is they want, if they could put their own narrative down on tape, that this would be a help to them.

For these nurses, every patient has a narrative, and preserving the narrative can become very important. We all tell stories, narratives that encapsulate the meaning of our lives. It is one way we explain our lives to ourselves. So as patients approach death, constructing and completing their narratives is a major task. Most of the nurses in this study believed that they had a duty to help their patients who wanted to review their lives.

Thus the nurses in this study operate on many different levels at once: the physical, social, cultural, and psychological. This "all at once" aspect of nursing, described by Paterson and Zderad (1988), is both the source of these nurses' pleasure and the source of their greatest tension. Nurses who practice holistically have to use their minds and their emotions, but they must not let either run away from them. They must be aware of their own reactions and they must be able to channel both faculties—head and heart—to the benefit of the patient.

In fact, feeling too much can run counter to nursing's goal and to the patient's health. Arthur R., who worked in an HIV unit where patients came back for treatment time and time again, described it this way:

> I was trying to explain to my assistant the other day that you cannot be emotionally involved, because then you might not make the proper decision. You might use your own defense mechanisms and say, "Well, this is happening, but it's really nothing," whereas it should be looked at. Or you might want to believe that everything's going to be fine, so you don't pick up on things, and then you're not doing the patient any good. And also, when they tell you, like this one guy said to me, "I want to stop everything," you might not be able to deal with that if you're emotionally involved. You might say, "Oh, don't talk like that," or "You're crazy," when actually the patient needs to talk to you. So you have to maintain a certain distance, you can't totally identify like it's your family or friends.

Achieving the proper relationship—not too close, not too distant—is not easy. Getting too close can mean the loss of critical distance so necessary if proper judgments are to be made. But too much distance may "trivialize distress" (Benner 1989) and prevent the formation of attachments. Balance is critical.

Nurses have to observe the people they are caring for without preconceptions and prejudices, but at the same time they must note ethnic, biological, religious, racial, sexual, economic, and social characteristics. They must be ready to admit similarities between themselves and those others who are different, yet they must be aware of what the differences mean, and how they affect the nurse-patient interaction. They try to feel close to their patients but they must be wary of overidentifying with them.

For the nurses in this study, the experience of work is emotionally draining, because so much that is different has to be absorbed and understood. Nursing is a total experience. It is also exhilarating because it offers practitioners an escape and a release from their own conventions of thought and behavior. By learning who the "other" is, they try on different ways of being human, and in the process, discover a wider range of human possibility for themselves.

Chapter 6
Ethical Dimensions of Care

The nurses in this study focus on the "other"; the patient is at the center of care. This focus creates a cognitive framework for resolving the ethical dilemmas they encounter in the care of HIV-infected patients. Most of these dilemmas center around questions of treatment, because HIV infection is not fully understood, and treatment is to some extent always problematic. The drugs used are very toxic, so there is always the possibility of serious side effects as well as the possibility of improvement. The nurses I interviewed relied on the principle that the patient should be the one to resolve the treatment dilemmas on the basis of informed consent.

When I asked the nurses in this study whether they faced any ethical dilemmas, most brought up the question of terminating treatment. As Nora J. described her experience:

> We have had questions like whether we should start feeding someone [providing nutrition intravenously] or not. We had one very bad situation here in our early days. This patient was being fed intravenously and he was dying under our eyes. He had diarrhea and diarrhea and diarrhea. There was nothing we could do. Everything we fed him passed right through. Yet I can see both sides of it. If a woman is dying, for example, and we give her feeding, we're prolonging her life for a period, and for all we know, maybe that's the most precious time the woman has. Maybe that's the time she would organize custody of her children. It's very difficult, but I think we have to be open and see how it goes on a case by case basis.

Nurses are not, by and large, in favor of aggressive treatment at any cost. This is certainly true for the nurses in this study, although they each fought long and hard to get their patients more time. A week at home, even if the patient eventually returned to the hospital, was a victory. But the nurses I interviewed believed that a point comes at which treatment no longer produces a benefit. When that point comes, care should begin to focus on making the patient comfortable.

This attitude can run counter to physicians' instincts. I was told, for instance, that some physicians will continue to recommend aggressive procedures such as lumbar punctures for patients at the final stages of HIV disease. The nurses I interviewed, however, because their attention is so firmly fixed on what is happening to the patient, are more ready to acknowledge the moment when treatment should logically stop. They are more ready to talk to patients about death than many of the physicians they work with. Many told me that they discussed death and dying with their patients. Emily B., practicing in home care, said it was always a question when a new infection cropped up or an old one flared again:

> I found that once I established my credibility with the patients, they would use me as a sounding board. They'd ask, "Should I do this treatment? Should I ignore these symptoms and let myself die?" If they developed a new infection, they always had to make the decision whether or not this would be the infection they would ignore and let kill them; so more than once I would be sitting there and having a discussion with somebody, "Well, you've got pneumonia, okay, what are you going to do about it?" And they would ask me very bluntly, "If I die of pneumonia, what's it going to be like?" I would explain that we'd order oxygen and control the symptoms. I'd explain we wouldn't let them lie there gasping for breath. We'd make them comfortable, because everybody is afraid it's going to be a painful process.

Helping patients choose the manner of their dying is a natural extension of these nurses' philosophy that their role is to look ahead for their patient, anticipate what is coming, and make provision for it. Thus these nurses will bring up the question of DNRs (Do Not Resuscitate orders), but they will do it in such a way that respects the patient's right to choose. Some patients will choose one thing, and some another. Stephanie C., who was particularly sensitive to the delicacy of the undertaking, explained how she approached the issue:

> Of course, some of them want to have every effort made to maintain life, and that's okay, too. As a health professional, I can put that hat on, and I can say, "Well, the better thing for you would be a DNR order," but the other part of me, as a nurse, says that the coping

mechanisms of the patient have to be respected. Some patients have denial to the last minute, to the last breath. Some patients tell you in an unwritten message, in a sort of metacommunication, that the way they want to die is to fight to the last minute, and not give up, and do everything possible to maintain life, and they want to be intubated [on an artificial ventilator]. That's okay if they want that, that's their choice if they want to die that way, just as long as they have the information there, so that they choose how they want to die. Right now, it's important to me that the patient has as much information as they need to make their choice. We tell them what it's like. The doctors are sometimes uncomfortable telling patients. Many of the jobs which are relegated to nurses are mop-up tasks, and one of the mop-up duties is to tell the patient what's really going to happen, what having KS of the lung means, which is that the tumor is going to grow and grow in spite of the chemotherapy, and eventually what will happen is that there will come a time when we will have to make a decision with the patient to intubate, and do everything possible to save him. I give patients the odds that they will never come off the machine. I come right out and say, "You'll spend two weeks of your life hooked to this as you die, or we can keep you comfortable and give you oxygen and comfort measures, and your family can be with you, and you can talk with them." It's really awful to be on a machine, but we try to be fair about the presentation. I think that many of them appreciate it. They say, "I never knew that, and let me think about it." Fine, we have time. I guess we're learning more and more to get to people earlier so they can make these decisions.

Gladys R. found that her young patients were more uncomfortable talking about DNRs than her older ones. She said:

A lot of the older patients don't mind signing the DNR. The younger ones really have to think about it. They really don't want to, because they think if they sign it nothing's going to be done for them, which is not true, but right away they say, "Oh, if I sign it, they're not going to feed me, they're not going to do anything for me," so they hem and haw; they don't want to sign it. So then when they get real sick, they just linger on and on and on until finally they go. But the old people they just relax and go.

It isn't only the patient who must be informed. Often the family has to be included also. And families have their own dynamics. As Gladys R. explained:

> If the patient can't do it [sign the DNR], the relatives often want to, but they're afraid to do it because they don't want to let the patient think that they don't care for them. Then you, the nurse, have to sit and explain to the family what it would be like for the patient. There are some [patients] that you would say, "No, leave him alone, no DNR for this one, you see a little bit of viability there," but there are others for whom it would only prolong the misery, so you don't want him put on a respirator. There are always some patients who look at other patients and they'll tell you they don't want to be on a machine. And then along comes a family member who says, "Do everything," and you say, "Well, the patient requested not to be put on the machine," but the family member insists. Then you're between a rock and a hard place.

The new New York State health proxy law is another option many nurses now raise with their patients. The law permits patients to nominate another person, not necessarily a relative, to make medical decisions for them if patients are unable to make a decision themselves.

These measures to ensure a dignified death, chosen by the patient, flow from a patient-centered approach to nursing in which the locus for decision-making is the patient. The nurse gives the patient as much information as he or she can, in a way that the patient can understand, but the final choice remains the patient's. This both reflects and supports these nurses' conception of nursing.

Many of these nurses see their role as helping their patients move comfortably from one state to another, whether that transition is from sickness to health or from sickness to death. Their goal is to help their patients make these transitions with as much dignity as possible. As Nora J. commented:

> I've had terrible experiences of having to attempt resuscitation on people who should have been allowed to die with dignity. That's the thing for me, having dignity. And that's the most horrific part of HIV disease for me, to see the way these people are slowly but surely stripped, inch by inch, of what is most important to them. I see patients who are three or four years older than me, and two months ago, they had a high-powered job downtown. Now this is happening to them. They have terrible diarrhea; they can't help themselves.

But the nurse is there to help the patient, as these nurses understand their role. They cannot make the disease disappear, but they can help the patient live more comfortably, and they anticipate, for the patient, what the next stage of the illness will require. This understanding of the nursing role often emerges gradually, as young nurses grow into experienced nurses. As Cassie N. said:

> When I first became a nurse, so many of my friends thought I was nuts, especially when I talked about my patients. I was so enthusiastic. When people asked me what I did, I said I saved lives for a living. But with AIDS patients, I can't say that. What I say now is that I help them maintain their quality of life for as long as possible. When that's no longer possible, I help ease them into the transition into death. That's what I have to say now. Because you don't save anyone with AIDS. You prolong their lives as long as possible, you keep them as comfortable as possible, you make them as well educated as possible about their disease, and when none of that is possible anymore, the only thing you have left is to keep them clean and comfortable on their way out. Help them make that transition. Help them decide how they want to be buried. Do they want to make a will? Do they want to contact people? Help them face these issues, if possible.

Such a conception of the nurse's role makes it easier to face death with acceptance, but it does not mean that having patients die is easy. As Stephanie C. said:

> It's very sad. For a while when you have a newly diagnosed patient, the struggle is to keep them healthy as long as possible, and that's great, and that works sometimes. Then sometimes out of a clear blue sky, unpredictably, a patient will come down with a very serious opportunistic infection, something that we hadn't foreseen, and will get extremely ill. The patient looks at me, and I look at them, and we both say to each other: "This is not fair. It's too soon."

Witnessing and not being able to prevent such suffering is hard to bear. As one nurse commented, "It's not death, it's the dying which is so hard to take." Once a patient is hospitalized with an opportunistic infection, nurses know that a first hospitalization will be followed by a second and a third. Bob G. described the disease as having "milestones": the diagnosis, the first medication, the first hospitalization, the wasting. Each of these milestones is a sign to the nurse of what is to come. Nurses watch their patients become shadows of their former selves, both physically and psychologically. Marilyn D. said this is very difficult:

> I've seen a lot of people who progressively, over a year, they get thinner and thinner with rashes and lesions and whatever. They

> really lose all of their well-being and they're just shells. Some were very vibrant, and that's sad, discouraging, really the hardest thing to watch. They just sort of fade away and become, at thirty or forty, walking around with a cane, like someone who is ninety.

Watching this deterioration is not easy. Nina H. said:

> I don't think death is the hardest thing in the world. I think a lot of the dying in between is. Patient after patient tells me that they have accepted the idea that they are going to die very soon. What they can't accept is losing control, or losing their independence, or losing their mind, or losing control of their bowels, or losing their friends who don't come to see them anymore. That's what I think people have a harder time with than death, and it's what I have a harder time with than death, to watch people go through that. There is a patient in the hospital right now who came in and was treated for PCP with a drug that can really cause a lot of damage to your pancreas. Well, first he got the side effects, and then what it caused is that now he's an insulin-dependent diabetic. So he got over his pneumonia and had to come back in the hospital for his diabetes. They got it under control and taught him how to do his insulin. He kind of appreciated the diabetes because it was a disease he could manage. He controlled his blood sugar pretty well, but now he's back in the hospital with CMV retinitis. It means he's going blind. He'd only been home about three weeks and now he's back in the hospital. He has to have a Hickman catheter [a permanent catheter for IV treatments] and daily infusions [of drugs] for the rest of his life. He has to have an IV infusion every day to prevent blindness, and just before all this he had limited his wants, his desires, to keeping his little studio apartment and not having it look like a hospital room. Now he's going to have a nurse coming all the time. He's going to have to have hospital equipment. He's going to have to have a home health-care attendant because he's really feeling overwhelmed. He really can't do it all, and all he wanted was to be able to stay home in his little place and not have it one big mess. But it's just one thing after another.

One infection is brought under control and another emerges. Quite often, treatment itself can produce the next problem. As Marcia B. said of one of her patients:

> I have one young man who's been doing extremely well for the past four years, and he has had six bouts of PCP and come through all of

> them with the same energy he went into them with. He does very well, but he has these bouts and in trying to control them they put a central line [permanent catheter] in, and every six weeks or so he gets several days of IV antibiotics to try to keep this PCP under control. He's done the aerosol bit and he still gets it back. Recently his central line got infected, and, in treating him with antibiotics, he became allergic to the first one. So they tried another, and he was allergic to that one. I have to go down to medical records today and pull out a list of all the antibiotics he's had to which he's become allergic, because the doctor wants him to wear a medical alert bracelet. We can't keep track any more. They've used practically everything under the sun on him. If he gets another infection I don't know what we're going to use.

Similar questions about when and how to treat cluster around female HIV-infected patients who are pregnant. It used to be thought that a majority of children born to HIV-infected women would contract HIV disease in utero, but this has been shown to be false. The infection rate is 20 to 50 percent (Bayer 1990; Thomas 1989). It was also thought that being pregnant would accelerate the course of HIV disease, but again this has not proved to be so (Novick et al. 1991).

So, although the most frequent medical advice for HIV-infected women is to either avoid becoming pregnant or to terminate the pregnancy, the chances of having a healthy baby are quite high. Sometimes, against many odds, choosing to continue a pregnancy has a happy ending. Carey M., who coordinates care for women in a perinatal HIV transmission study, told the following story:

> We took care of a woman who came to New York to get medical care for her two-year-old who had AIDS. Her husband was in Brazil dying of AIDS, and she was HIV positive but not sick yet. She was pregnant when she arrived, and in her eighth month, she had PCP. While she was in the hospital with PCP, her two-year-old died, and she went out on pass to the funeral. It was the most incredibly heartbreaking thing. She had this kid [the one who died] who was neurologically impaired and the mother really cared for that child, and she was pregnant, and we all sort of went through it with her. She was really religious, and we went through her agony over whether to have an abortion or not, and she finally decided she had to keep the baby. She's one of the few people that I really believed that it was for spiritual reasons or religious. Most of the time people say it and you find out they had two abortions previously. She was a person we really watched go through her own spiritual struggle over this. She

> had the baby, and found out a week or two later that her husband had died in Brazil. It was just dramatic, talk about courage, and her little baby is two-years-old now, and she is not infected.

Nurses have to keep in mind that this can happen, at the same time that they recognize that this outcome is not guaranteed. Other patients may not be so lucky. But again it is not for the nurse to tell the patient what to do.

A further complication with pregnant women who are HIV-infected is the question of whether to put them on AZT, which, at the time of this study, was the only federally approved drug for HIV disease. AZT may help the mother, but there is no definitive information yet about its effect on the fetus. Similar problems surround the prescription of Bactrim for PCP prophylaxis. What may be good for the mother may harm the fetus. In the absence of certainty, the nurses in this study who cared for mothers and newborns left the final decision to the mother.

This is a different perspective from that of many physicians, whose instincts are to recommend action and therapy (Payer 1988). These instincts rest on a desire to treat and cure, but the nurses in this study believed that this desire should be modified to fit the patient's situation. Alice D., who has over thirty years of experience in hospitals and private practice, explained why she thought some physicians resisted recognizing when the moment to cease treatment arrived:

> I think physicians' mind set is that they want to cure people, or they want to delay the dying as long as they can, and that's a noble and admirable quality. I wouldn't want it any other way. But I think sometimes they lose sight of the fact that sometimes they're almost causing more discomfort. Where's the scale of balance? How much do you try to delay the progress of the disease, when at the same time, you're decreasing the quality of life of that person? How do you do that and try to maintain some kind of quality of life? Here I think informed consent is important. You make decisions with the patients. Some patients will say, "Look, do what you have to do. I'll put up with the nausea and the vomiting and the diarrhea and whatever. I want to hang in there, because who knows, tomorrow there might be a cure and I want to be around for it." Whereas other patients will say, "Look, this is not a life; this is no way to live."

Accepting the patient's decision is not simple and automatic. It means that the nurse must listen not only to what patients say but also to the patients' mood as they say it. A patient may state that they want to stop treatment, but the nurse cannot accept such a statement uncritically. It must be interpreted in the light of what else the nurse knows about the patient. As Phyllis H. said:

> I think that the patient has the ultimate say, but you have to be real careful that they understand all the implications. One patient who looked like he was going to die said to me, "I feel so bad, I don't even want to take the medication. Why bother? I should just die." And I said to him, "Well, I know what you're feeling, and I guess you could do that, you have the power to do that, but we just diagnosed this new problem you have, and there's medication for it, so why not try it? Why don't you try to take the medication, because you might feel better?" He did and he felt a little bit better, not a whole lot better, but he did feel better and he stopped losing weight. So, yeah, I made an ethical decision. I could have said, "Okay, go ahead, do what you want." But I said, "You still have a chance here, I think you owe it to yourself to try." I felt he was depressed, and when you're depressed, you need somebody to pull you and say, "No, don't just stay home, come out to a movie." That's why I said, "I think you should try this before you give up."

Clarifying the choices, giving the patient all the information that will facilitate an informed opinion, being honest without being brutal—these are all part of the nurse's responsibilities. Each patient represents a different set of possible outcomes. As Gladys R. said:

> We've had many patients whom we intubated and they got better and could even go home. I'd say to them, "You know there isn't enough oxygen circulating in your body. In order for you to go home, we have to intubate you; you'll be on a machine, just don't fight it." They're fully conscious, so when you have to intubate them, it's the devil, because no medication [sedative] takes properly. So you talk to them and say, "Remember I told you this is a tube, don't pull it out, because if you pull it out, then you won't make it. In order for you to make it, you have to have it." There are some you can't say that to. You don't want to lie to them, which we don't. But sometimes it's hard. They're young. These young men cry; they haven't lived their lives. It's hard for us and hard for them.

Difficulties also arise over pain relief for patients. According to these nurses, many of the physicians they work with are reluctant to prescribe large amounts of pain medication. They are concerned about addiction and about the possibility that opiates can depress a patient's breathing, bringing death a little sooner than otherwise.

One nurse described a patient with brain lesions who was on a morphine drip for many weeks before he died. The psychiatrist on the unit was very uncomfortable with the length of time the patient had the drip; he was afraid the morphine would kill him. But the patient was very afraid of going mad, and he did seem demented on occasion. There were times when he did not recognize his lover. Without the morphine, he would often pace the halls in an agitated state. The morphine drip kept him comfortable and calm, but conscious. Eventually, the psychiatrist began to see it the nurse's way; the morphine was not killing the patient. The dosage never got so high that his breathing was depressed. But the morphine took the edge off his anxiety and he had a peaceful end.

Sometimes, however, there seems to be a callous disregard for patients' suffering. One nurse, trained in Europe, was upset by the agonized deaths she witnessed on her unit. She said many patients did not receive enough pain medication and so died in great pain. There is no need for anyone to die this way, but it does happen. Stephanie C. described an episode in the pediatric unit which she felt should never have happened:

> A little boy I remember, a three-year-old boy, who was in great pain. I know that he was in great pain; he was dying of AIDS. We had his crib full of stuffed toys. He loved stuffed toys. He had so many he was actually lying on them. His mother and father abandoned him, and so he became ours. We used to get him out in the wheelchair, and he would whimper. His belly got so big, it was his liver. Everything was going wrong with him, and so I got them to give him some oral morphine, by drops. They gave him the oral morphine, and I will never forget this, the neurologist came up the next day and said, "Don't drug this kid, the child's not in pain." And, in the meantime, when we would pick him up under the arms to put him into the wheelchair, he would scream. . . . We had known this child from the beginning, from the first time he walked through the door. So we watched him progressively get sicker and sicker, and we knew when he was in pain. We knew that it was not like him to sit there and say, "Uh, uh, uh," that kind of thing. It was true that the child would nap on the morphine. He would doze, but after a while this effect wears off, after the body adjusts. At any rate, the neurologist didn't like that, he was the chief of neurology, so he said, "I want you to cut out the morphine and I don't want this child drugged; this child's going to live a long time, etc. etc." So all the doctors said, "The chief said that, you know." And they cut out the morphine and the child died in agony after two days.

But for this nurse there was a lesson in the tragedy. She used the episode to avert similar incidents. As she said:

> I talked until I was blue in the face, but the pediatricians were all frightened of crossing the hierarchy. They didn't want to start trouble, but you see, this is not going to happen again. I will not let it happen again. I will remind them of this. I will use it as ammunition, so that this child who died in agony, it is not going to happen again. We should learn from him; he was a good teacher. He taught us a lot. Let's not do this again. So I will fight like a tiger for the next child who is in pain. That child will go out sedated.

These nurses see themselves as the patients' advocates. In order to be the patient's advocate, however, a nurse has to know the patient well, and this is something which HIV disease makes possible. Because HIV-infected patients have frequent hospital admissions and need continual care in various settings, they are well known to their nurses.

Many nurses said that the pleasure of patient contact was something they sought and something they found with HIV-infected patients because of the numerous hospital admissions and treatments these patients needed. As Gladys R. said:

> [In other units] they go off into the sunset. . . . But [in the AIDS unit] it was like family. It was family. We used to sit in the room with the patient. They'd be watching TV and we'd be sitting there writing in the chart. And we could observe them, because I could be writing and then I'd look up and then I'd write again, and look up, and I could see exactly what was going on, because you take care of them, you bathe them, you set them up, and after lunch is when you'd sit down and write charts. You'd sit in the room and you'd write, and then you could observe anything that was going on. If there was a change, they'd change right in front of your eyes.

Gladys found the sense of community in HIV care which she had enjoyed in the early days of the dialysis unit.

Familiarity is essential if the nurse is to understand the HIV-infected patient. It is a kind of relationship neither so easy to achieve with other patients, nor so necessary. As Robin M. said:

> I did critical care for many years and there is no ongoing relationship with the patients. That's why I chose it, I wanted to be technical. I wanted to look at the monitor and I wanted to do this high-tech stuff, like someone comes in with a heart attack, and I jump in and do my

> heart massage, and defribilate them, and I save them. It was a lot of action, and I liked it, and I still really like that action, and I miss it a bit. But on the other hand, I never had to think so much about any patient's lifestyles or where they come from. The main thing was they should not be in danger. There was a lot of counseling and telling them what to do and not to do, but they would leave and I would not know who they were anymore. But here everything stays with you.

For many nurses this personal relationship with patients is why they went into nursing and why they stay in it. It is also the cause of a great deal of tension. The nurse wants to be connected to the patient, to be understanding, to do what the patient wants, or to do what will help the patient. But often, and particularly with the HIV-infected patient, the needs of the patient, especially the emotional needs, can be a source of conflict. As Marcia B. explained:

> I can think of someone who's on the unit right now who I feel is extremely needy, and a lot of it is really an intense loneliness. There are people who feel extremely lonely and I think that's the most difficult thing to manage [for a nurse]. It's almost like, no matter what you do, you see that patient, and you start to feel guilty because you haven't met that need. So I think that's what makes nurses draw back. They say, "I know you want me there, but I'm doing something else," and then they feel guilty. It's easy then to think, "I don't like you [the patient] very much," or "I don't want to be around you any more." I can understand that, that some people are so overwhelmingly needy. Sometimes it helps, it depends on the patient of course, but there are some patients you can say this to: "I want to be here for you, and I recognize that you are lonely. I want to spend time with you, and I feel bad I can't make it all go away for you, but I have to go take care of other patients, and I'm afraid you're still going to be lonely when I leave." To acknowledge the way you feel helps the patient, and I think it helps the nurse as well, instead of just trying to give what you can and run away and feel kind of bad about it. But there are definitely some patients you pull back from.

Some nurses felt badly that they pulled back from patients, and that they pulled back from patients at the end, when they felt the patient needed them most. But it was important that they preserve their own sense of self even when they wanted to act otherwise. One nurse said:

> You see someone coming, he's PCP, first admission. Okay, it's very easy because it's nothing threatening, but you see him at the end of the disease, when you've known this guy for maybe eighteen months or a year. You see him disintegrating, and there's nothing left. There's only a shell of what you knew before. And it's very hard to reach out to that person. It might just be me, it might be just a personal issue with me, but I don't think so. I think it's more than me that sometimes, when someone is so sick, it's so hard to reach out. You may want to, but to be able to is another thing.

Another nurse agreed. She said:

> I sometimes distance myself if I've become attached to somebody. I spend less time in their room. There are ways of doing it. I recognize that. I had one patient who just died who was one of those people; when they come into the hospital, the chemistry is just right. His wife was lovely and he had two young girls. Then his wife said, "I'm going to take him home [to die]." Which she did, magnificently. Well, they lived near me, but I never said we were neighbors. As it happened, I saw her in church, and she came up to me afterward and said, "I didn't know you lived here." And she asked if I would come see her husband. I said, "Sure," but I didn't go because I really loved him. And as it happened, a couple of days before he died, his wife called and said that her husband was really bad, so I went to see him the next day. He was barely conscious but he did recognize me, and I said, "I'm so happy to see you," and he said, "Same here." Then his wife called the next morning and said he was dying. There was a definite case where I did hold back, because I can't tell you how it hurts.

Another nurse had exactly the opposite problem. She found herself becoming too close to her patients and had difficulty maintaining distance. She envied nurses who could maintain boundaries. As she said:

> Being in administration is safer for me, although I loved bedside nursing. The costs were too high, at least for doing it all the time. I'm one of these all or nothing people, and that tends to get in your way a lot. I would have drawn back [from patients] if I could have. I'm at the other end of the spectrum from the nurse who can't control pulling back. I can't control the investment. The other, if I could have had my druthers, I would have preferred that. Maybe there's a

> cost to the patient there [in pulling back], but I'm not sure there isn't a cost to the patient also with the nurse who overinvests herself. That's something I recognize.

Patient and nurse must make contact but neither must invade the other. Empathy and receptivity move the patient and nurse toward each other, but each must be careful not to overwhelm the other. Sometimes in fact they need to defend themselves from the other. Thus in one sense they are together, and in another they are apart (Havens 1986).

The cumulative effect of caring for HIV-infected patients can be depression and despair when there is so much to be done and so much to feel. It is difficult to keep on providing care while coping with the intellectual and emotional demands of the disease, the patients, and other caregivers. What many nurses report is that, after holding up for a long time, the death or deterioration of a particular patient triggers a strong reaction. As Emily D. said:

> It's funny how it snowballs. I took care of [HIV-infected] people for years and I was functioning just fine. Then there was a group of people I got particularly close to, for whatever reason you always identify more with some people than with others. I lost three of these patients in one week. All of them were long-term people, like upwards of two years. One was expected to die, one chose to die, and he was all prepared, but one was totally unexpected. I got to the home, and the lover answered the door; he had come home for lunch and found him dead. That was horrible. In the third case, the sister was the caregiver and she was clinging to him to the point of absurdity, but he was feeding on it. This guy had KS everywhere. He was all swollen. His legs were swollen, his scrotum was swollen, he was miserable. He was on morphine round the clock and he was still miserable. Yet he couldn't let go to die. She wouldn't let him go. It was totally unbearable. It was gruesome. He was suffering too. Then he died finally, and what happened to me was I hadn't let myself mourn any of the other losses, and it all came crashing down on me, and I started to cry for everyone.

The emotional strains of nursing, particularly nursing a new and infectious disease, demand great self-control from nurses. They have to be able to temper their responses, both toward and away from the patient. They have to be sympathetic, but not too sympathetic. They have to be clinical, but not solely clinical. Nurses don't want to shortchange their patients, but at the same time they need to retain their independence and their autonomy.

One way these nurses find to do this is to laugh, to find the humor in the day's events. Laughter assuages the pain and the feelings that are a daily part of caring for HIV-infected patients. Gladys R. commuted to work with a colleague and described their trip home in the evenings: "I guess we keep our sanity by laughing, traveling in the car going home. We replay the day going home, with the different incidents. We just laugh like crazy. I guess people see us in the car laughing and probably say, 'Look at those two crazy women.' Sometimes patients are so funny, you have to laugh."

Most nurses, when asked, will say that the personal connection with their patient is central to their practice. It is, certainly for the nurses in this study, the avenue through which they achieve their nursing goals and their professional and personal satisfaction. Yet that personal connection contains the seeds of many conflicts. In order to resolve conflicts with due regard to each party's interests, nurses have to have a developed sense of themselves, as well as an understanding of their patients as individuals. Establishing the proper boundaries is essential; once established, nurse and patient can begin to develop a mutually satisfying relationship. As Gladys R. remarked:

> Some of the patients, they're street persons, but, once you calm them down, most won't curse at you, though of course some still will. And you say to them, "You keep it up and you go out of here." They walk off and mumble under their breath, or go in and slam the door and curse at you behind the door. You don't pay them any mind because they're behind the door. Then they come out and they say, "Miss ———, may I have some medicine? Give it to me." And I say, "I didn't hear the word 'please.'" Then they say, "Oh, may I have some, please?" You constantly have to be like a mother, you have to constantly train them. But sometimes, like I'll be going up ——— Avenue, and someone will say, "Hi," and of course I keep right on walking, but then they'll say, "Nurse, hi," and sometimes they holler, "Hello, Miss ———." They wave like we're old friends. They come to clinic and they come to look for me on the floor, or they send a message. "Tell Miss ——— to come see me." And of course I go. One of them was in the clinic and he told them I was his mother, and they searched the whole hospital for me. He was a prisoner. He couldn't come look himself. But I like that, when they remember me.

Chapter 7
Making a Difference: Personal and Professional Growth

The Rewards of Caring for HIV-Infected Patients

Nursing that takes into account every facet of a patient's life is difficult work, so it is not surprising that many of the nurses I talked with entertain from time to time thoughts of leaving nursing. One said, "Every Friday I think about quitting." Some actually have left nursing and then come back, because there are rewards in nursing that they cannot find in other occupations. Carol H. stated forthrightly, "All of us do this because we get something out of it." And Carey M. said:

> Sometimes I say I want to open up a fast food store in the country, but I think what still sustains me is the fact that I am doing something for humanity in whatever small way it can be done. And it's not just what I know how to do but the fact that I choose to do it. That's the satisfaction, knowing that I'm doing something really important and perhaps providing for a group of people something they wouldn't have otherwise.

Most of the nurses I interviewed described their work as "important" and "worthwhile." It is important because it deals with serious issues, with life and death, with illness and health, with hope and despair. In addition, HIV disease is *the* medical crisis of our time and through their care of patients with HIV disease, these nurses are part of an experience unique to the last decade of the twentieth century.

HIV care is worthwhile because the nurse can effect improvement and change. Although there is no cure, the treatments for opportunistic infections have improved greatly since the early 1980s. Nurses now have the satisfaction of being able to alleviate many problems. As Stephanie C. said in a second interview, "Now at least we can make certain predictions; we know what helps and what doesn't." She went on to say:

> I think we're getting better at picking up a lot of disease processes. We're much more aware of what can happen now, so that we can act prescriptively. We know that when a patient's T-cells get to be below two hundred, we know then that they are liable for a lot of things, for example, TB. We expect pulmonary TB. If they haven't had TB before, they're probably going to get it now. So if they haven't had a chest X-ray in the last six months, we send them down for one. We become hypervigilant at that point. And we also tell the patient, "Look, at this point in the disease process, you can expect some infections. Here's what you can expect." I think that takes a lot of the fear out of the process. It can be overwhelming. For example, the patient comes into the ER with a 105-degree temperature. The family doesn't understand; they think the patient's going to die right there. The patient too thinks, "Well, this is it." Now, if we told the patient before, "You're going to get very high fevers and feel that you can't lift your head off the pillow; you're going to ache all over," then they're all somewhat prepared for what's going to happen. We're doing better teaching, better counseling, and better treatment. We're maintaining patients on a plateau longer. We're shutting off that AIDS period, keeping it at bay as long as possible. We're getting better at it, so that's good.

Thus, on the first and simplest level, the rewards of doing this kind of nursing begin with the patient's reaction. If the patient feels more comfortable, if he or she appreciates the effort the nurse is making and expresses that appreciation, nurses know that they are doing a good job. As Emma J., in charge of patient care for HIV-infected patients in a suburban hospital, said:

> Everybody smiles when I walk in the room. I get satisfaction out of being one of the few people they are able to talk to and confide in. I'm someone who can perhaps give them some comfort or some help in a world that is just beating up on them. The satisfaction I get is that really I have not found anybody who is not happy to see me. When I walk into the room everyone says, "Oh, I'm glad you're here." That's enough.

Such a response from patients can be a boost to a nurse's self-esteem. It can make the hours and struggles all worthwhile. As Bette V. said:

> Personally, to me, there are great rewards in it. It's wonderful to your ego lots of times. People are so appreciative, and so sweet, especially AIDS patients on the whole. Many of them, perhaps they've been places where they weren't taken care of well, or they've heard stories about not being taken care of well, and they appreciate the least little thing.

For these nurses, most of whom remember the disdain with which nursing was viewed until quite recently, expressions of appreciation are sweet indeed.

In addition, being able to do it right, and being able to do it for people who don't expect it, can be a pleasure in itself. For Maria J., whose patients were all IV drug users or the partners of IV drug users, it is this aspect of nursing that keeps her going:

> Patients tell me, "I'm glad I met you." They will say they never had anyone care for them. The patients here don't have families. They've used drugs and everyone has disowned them. Or women have been infected by people who used drugs and they still disown them. People here don't ordinarily seek medical care. They tell me I make a difference. Just when I think, "Oh, I don't know if I can continue to do this," then I hear something like that and I say I have to continue. I have to because I think I make a difference.

This phrase, "making a difference," recurs frequently when these nurses talk about the satisfactions of nursing HIV-infected patients. It seems like a shorthand code that expresses both the difficulties under which they work and the goals they seek. They do not aspire to greatness; their aim is to do what they can—it is an aim that will be limited by the constraints of the health-care system, by their own capacities, and by their patients' responses.

Yet they know that what they are doing is important and does make a difference, even if it's only with a small group of patients or within one hospital. Particularly for nurses in the municipal hospital system, where resources are limited and the patients have multiple problems, the knowledge that, without their care, these patients would be in even direr straits sustains and rewards them. As Gretchen S., who worked in a busy and somewhat chaotic municipal clinic, said:

> Every patient who comes through that door is not someone with nothing else to do but go to the hospital. People here are for the most part extremely ill, in terrible circumstances. We have to pick up the pieces, so to speak. I stay here, I guess, because I feel needed here

> more than at another hospital. Here there's such a glaring need, and luckily I'm a member of a team of people who are very dedicated and who make working a joy, even though the work's very difficult.

Nina H. agreed. She said: "I know people are going to die, but if I can make a difference in someone's death, then I've made a difference. If that person who is dying knows that they are not dying alone, and if I can hold their hand while they go, then I've done something."

In addition to the pleasure of helping another, there is the attraction, for many of these nurses, of coming face to face with existential mysteries of human life. As one nurse said, "There are universal themes, there are commonalities in all of this." Nursing HIV-infected patients puts caregivers in touch with fundamental questions of human existence, particularly how to live in a world where death is inevitable. For many of these nurses, therefore, HIV nursing is an opportunity to consider, *in their work,* what living and dying mean. For them, part of the satisfaction of HIV care is helping patients face death, as well as facing the possibility of death themselves. Lore H., who was about to return to bedside nursing of HIV-infected patients after some time in administration, said:

> One of the things that I think sets people who work in AIDS apart—I know it sets me apart, I can only imagine that it sets other people apart—is, if you talk with people who work in business or you talk with people who work in almost any field, and you talk about life being short, that old cliché, and you talk about what's important and why things are important and stuff, their work is very shallow and doesn't have as much meaning as mine.

Caring for HIV-infected patients can also put nurses in touch with much that is admirable in people's lives, particularly in individual's and families' responses to the illness. In this there are similarities to caring for cancer patients, especially as this care took form twenty years ago when there was little to be done for patients. Then as now, the heroism some patients and families exhibited could be an inspiration to their caregivers. As Carey M. said of her observations of women and children with HIV disease: "The poignancy of some of the families and the courage I see demonstrated is remarkable, and I suppose that being allowed to be close to that is to be privileged. When I talk about it, I'm very close to tears."

Taking care of HIV-infected patients lets nurses get close to some of the worst and some of the best that human beings are capable of. Some HIV-infected patients display everything that is despicable in human behavior; others are truly heroic. Alice D. was particularly struck by the selflessness many of her patients showed by participating in clinical trials:

> I've been really impressed, particularly with the gay population, how they have been willing to experiment with all these drugs, knowing that it is never going to help them. It's not going to cure them, but it may help someone else down the road. They have to come in and have their blood drawn and various other things that are not terribly pleasant. And it could be easy for them to say, "To heck with it, I'm going to live as comfortably as I can. I'm not going to subject myself to all that." But many of them really have a very altruistic outlook on things.

Nurses taking care of mothers and children are particularly struck by the fortitude and endurance they witness. Carey M., who was a member of a team studying the transmission of HIV disease from mother to child, said of one of her patients:

> I think of the young woman of thirty who just recently died. She was already blind from a genetic disorder, and she had a kid also to take care of. I was just totally amazed at her ability to cope. Actually, what strikes me most about the patients I work with is their incredible ability to live with this. Their courage astounds me. I think of another patient who is very sick and weak and thin—she's repeatedly getting different things, and it's very sad to see. But she's also partaken of everything around her. She got help from GMHC [Gay Men's Health Crisis], she got a buddy, she got everything she could get as far as social services, she got herself the best medical treatment she could, she got herself into Sloan Kettering [New York City's preeminent hospital for cancer patients], and she's made arrangements for her daughter's care. Her family's coming up to get to know the little girl so that when she does die, her daughter will know them.

Some patients change their lives dramatically when they become ill, showing their nurses that transformation is possible. Alice D. commented:

> I've heard people say so many times, "Now that I'm dying, my life has never been so good." The quality of their life, the way they've kind of reconstructed their whole way of looking at things, has changed, and it's really increased their inner peace, their strength, their spirituality, their way of coping with things. I think it's interest-

ing that, faced with such a grim prognosis, people can still find some kind of meaning to their lives, and still maintain a positive attitude. They decide who their real friends are, the quality of the time they spend with them becomes so much more meaningful. So it's not all bad, so it's not all grim. I've gotten a lot of very positive things from them. I suppose it's like any terminal disease, you learn not to take anything off of anybody. You learn not to mess with the petty things of life and you really find out what your priorities are.

In this scenario, the patient becomes the teacher. Nurses learn from their patients. One nurse who headed a hospital clinic said of her patients:

> It is amazing how patients support one another. We have a large Hispanic population. Most of these patients are homosexual, while our black male population is mostly IVDUs. Gradually our female population is growing, mixed between sex partners and IVDUs, but across risk and cultural differences, support is given. One group helped a female patient get to church every Sunday. Others visit "clinic friends" when they are hospitalized.

Some of the instruction from patients is about the right way to provide humane clinical care. As Stephanie C. said:

> I had a wonderful patient who was a lovely man; I'll never forget him. I learned so much from him. He had a nice death. He did not want to be intubated. He had cancer, KS, and it went to his lungs. So he was struggling to breathe, and he didn't want to be resuscitated; so what we did was set up morphine shots around the clock so that he would be sedated. His family was there and now what I have is this imprint of ——— in my mind, and when I see a patient who has a similar problem, I then can take that and put it right into practice.

What taking care of HIV-infected patients does for many of these nurses is enlarge their own understanding of human problems. It also increases the number of different responses they can offer their patients. Because the questions patients ask frequently have no easy answers, this process can become a collaborative one, in which nurses and patients approach problems together. Stephanie C. described the process in this way:

> For example, take a young woman who is minding her own business, who is not taking drugs, who is not doing anything, and all of a

> sudden, she gets the news that she's HIV positive. Then comes a series of infections and this downward slippery slope, and she might say to me, "I know I'm going to die, how can I do this with as much dignity and grace as possible?" And I don't know, I don't know. I'm using the inventory I have as a person, and there are times when I feel that I don't have enough to be a resource to these women. What I do in those instances is tell the women, "I'm here for you, we'll explore this thing together, and as much as I can, I won't leave you. We'll solve the problems together, and we'll do as much as we can together. And whatever we learn together, we will teach other women."

Thus individual experience is preserved and incorporated into knowledge that is available to others. Nursing becomes something more than analyzing a patient's condition and applying the appropriate remedy. It becomes a creative process between the nurse and patient. And what is learned is then brought to other patients.

Nurses learn from patients and patients learn from nurses—not only about HIV disease and how to treat it, but about human relations and tolerance. In order to do this, nursing practitioners have to be open and tolerant, and one of the rewards of this nursing is to see families and other personnel develop similar attitudes. George N. said:

> I like to see people have time to resolve some of their internal and external problems, to see families accept certain things. I'm not saying it's something they want to accept, but it's something that society as a whole doesn't want to accept. For some families to come to the realization that, "Yes, this is the person's lifestyle, and we're going to accept that," and "Yes, this may or may not have led to their death, but they're mine to take care of, regardless of what I think about this." This has some satisfaction. For instance, you may get a substance abuser who has been completely disengaged from his family for many, many years, and in the course of his exploits may have produced two or three children, and he seems completely alone. But you will find that there are children and loved ones, and sometimes you're able to get a family some assistance so that the children can come to say goodbye. You work everything out, the legal paperwork, and the children say goodbye, and that's satisfaction, that the patient could live long enough to have that.

Nurses who organize such reconciliations know they are having a real impact on patient's lives, even if it's only at the end of life. It is one of the satisfactions these nurses report. And part of the reason nurses enjoy this work is that they can have an impact greater than in other specialties. There is considerable scope here for nurses' initiative and intervention. All sorts of problems have to be addressed and all sorts of skills are needed. Nurses are fully engaged. For some, it becomes an opportunity to be the kind of nurse they always wanted to be. As Emma J. said:

> I've just moved to a clinician position, but I'm still there to help with morning care if they bog down. I can pitch in and give a bath or change a bed, or whatever, but my primary focus is different. What they really want is for me to spend more time with the people in scatter [not in dedicated AIDS unit] beds, give them more emotional support. I'm very free. If I go in and somebody is having a really bad day, I can sit there for a good long time. Nobody is going to pressure me. That's a gift. And it's all the things that you ever wanted to do, that you were told good nurses did, but you never had time to do.

Caring for HIV-infected patients allows these nurses to realize the idealistic goals that drew them to nursing from the start. The lower patient-nurse ratio prevailing in most dedicated HIV units gives nurses the time to get to know their patients. The fact that other health-care providers are not competing for these patients gives nurses a freer hand and a chance to organize care on nursing principles. Because of the nature of the illness, the patient populations, whether in hospital or not, need the comprehensive involvement that these nurses see as key to their concept of nursing.

Nursing is central to the management of HIV disease; thus, in HIV care, nurses find their skills, their attitudes, and their performance validated and approved. This contrasts nicely with the wholesale denigration of their profession that occurred during the 1970s, partly as a consequence of the women's movement, when traditional female occupations such as nursing and teaching lost status and respect.

In addition, the nurses I interviewed have found that being the nurse they always wanted to be holds numerous personal rewards. They enjoy the gratitude of their patients. They know they are doing something that is important to another person and that gives them pleasure. They help their patients achieve a better understanding of how to make the most of life, and in the transformations that they witness and support, nurses share in their patients' courage and fortitude.

With their patients, they face both the griefs and joys attendant on mortality, and they change themselves through their involvement with others who are also changing. Along with their patients, they can experience rebirth and renewal. They move with their patients from one discovery to another. They participate in their patients' progress.

This progress is toward a more profound understanding of the human condition. What nurses learn on this journey they bring to other patients. They share with others the knowledge they have gained through their acute and sympathetic observation of and involvement with their patients.

Thus the narratives these nurses retain and the ones they want to share are about the successes they experience in caring for HIV-infected patients, because it is in these successes that they experience growth and renewal. Essential to these successes is the personal connection nurses establish with their patients, because their successes are dependent on the relationship of trust and respect that they create with the patient.

Personal Growth and Development

Nurses have to study their patients carefully in order to establish this relationship of trust and respect, and the process through which they come to understand their patients is conducive to their own growth and development. As Stephanie C. said:

> Patients grow with you and you grow with them. It's a learning process. What I try to do is take from each patient, and I carry what I've learned into the next situation. It's a reciprocal process that takes place between the patient and myself, whereby we sort of help each other as we go along and enlighten each other.

In caring for HIV patients, many accepted attitudes and assumptions become subject to scrutiny. In order to do this work, nurses must be aware of and willing to examine their own beliefs about social life, sexuality, drug use, and other issues usually hidden behind the scrim of conventional thought and behavior. HIV care therefore can be an opportunity for personal development because, when cultural expectations are disturbed, insightful self-examination can be the route back to equilibrium. Having to confront that which, until now, was hidden or denied, such as racial, ethnic, class, or sexual differences, makes nurses rethink their social world. As Nora J. said:

> Have I grown in this work? Definitely. I've obtained a wealth of knowledge, all sorts of knowledge. From going to various conferences, I've met people from all over the world and the U.S., which has definitely increased my growth and knowledge. I've worked with

people from all different populations, and it's been interesting psychologically and emotionally, particularly in working with prison populations. I've learned a lot about areas I normally wouldn't have learned about, about patients' families, about how they want to care for the patient at home, about social services. I know more about human nature and what goes on with people, whether they're in a higher economic class or a lower one.

This process can force nurses to develop technical skills they might not have needed in another kind of nursing. Chris T., whose position as an AIDS advocate brought her into contact with high-level government officials, said:

I think my experience with AIDS and the jobs that I've had have allowed me to advance and develop in areas that I know I otherwise wouldn't have gotten into, for example, public speaking. I'm not the best public speaker, but I can do it, and five or seven years ago, I would never have thought I could. I've done a fair amount of it now. Getting involved with computers and research and data stuff, that's also been a part of it. I'm not expert in that but it's a learning thing, something to add to your skills. Along the way, with AIDS, I've been pulled and pushed to advance some of my skills, like writing and management skills.

Many of the nurses I interviewed said that taking care of HIV-infected patients changed them. On a day-to-day level, they are less concerned with trivialities. As one nurse wrote in response to the survey:

For a long time I maintained that it [nursing HIV patients] had little or no effect on me except to make me more sensitive to issues of death and dying. I now realize that indeed, there have been some very long-term effects. I appreciate family and friends more than I used to. I have also ended an unsatisfactory marriage because I realize that life and time are too precious to waste. I don't believe in the hereafter; therefore I think that this life should be lived to the fullest. Dealing with AIDS has made me more appreciative of life. I try to pass this appreciation on to my family, friends, and particularly my children.

Gretchen S. agreed:

I do think that there's been a lot of personal growth in terms of this idea of my work, my clinical work being a creative thing, and so

> somehow I've got more of a focus on today. This is what we've got. I'm not a religious person, but this is what we have here. And this should be good. We should make it good because we don't know what it's going to be. Sometimes it's hard to remember, but it's really become a philosophy that I've tried to keep in mind as I go through the day. If it's sunny out, just be glad it's sunny out. If it rains, look at something else, look at shapes, look at figures. I'm not going to take my pleasures in ten years. Also I want my interactions [with other people] to be real; I don't really have time for most mundane chitchat.

The central issue that nurses caring for HIV-infected patients have to face and accept is the issue of their own mortality. In order to care for HIV-infected patients, nurses must understand their feelings about death, their own and others'. As one nurse said, "Having people die all around you opens up the box; you have to examine your own mortality." Accepting death as a part of life is central to HIV care. As Carey M. said: "The biggest issue is confronting my own mortality. There's no escaping that. That comes up daily, several times a day, with patients and with families. I guess it's made me get in touch with my philosophical self." Nora J. put it rather differently: "In order to do this work you have to be convinced of your own immortality."

And indeed almost all the nurses I interviewed believed that there was something after death. Some believed in the Christian traditions of heaven and hell, but the majority embraced vaguer images of another life. Bette V. said:

> I guess my own feeling is that there is a continuum of experience that includes life and death, and so it's a sort of spiral. That doesn't mean that my focus isn't on living. It's very important to get whatever we can, whatever experiences we can out of our lives, rather than focus on what's coming afterward, but to recognize also that there will be something afterward.

Carey M. commented:

> I'm not sure there's a conventional heaven, but I think there is something after death. I feel it when people say to me, "Oh, I wish I'd said that to my mother or sister or whoever, my loved one, before he or she died," and I say, "That's all right, you're saying it now and he or she knows it." My way of getting through someone's death is to say, "I bet you're somewhere." I talk to them. I don't have a clear idea

> of what it's like, but I believe that there is some collective, unconscious something there.

Whatever conclusions these nurses come to, what is important is that caring for HIV-infected patients encourages them to think about personal mortality and to come to some peace with the prospect of dying. Much as many of their patients do, they discover, through their involvement with HIV disease, some of their real beliefs about the conundrums of human life. The ability of these nurses to do this hinges on their openness not only to their patients but to themselves. Nurses must monitor their own reactions as well as those of their patients. They have to face, within themselves, the same fears that their patients face, and they have to resolve them, as many of their patients resolve them, in order to continue their work.

As these nurses move toward greater self-knowledge, they find confirmation of who they think they are or hope to be in the reflections others mirror back to them. The first image reflected back to them is from their patients. Sometimes they are surprised at what their patients see. Toby B. was startled by how she appeared to one of her patients:

> His lover had been here, and this patient used to come in to visit. They were lovely. I used to talk to them and joke with them, but he was always very businesslike, and he did a lot of business on the phone while he was visiting his lover. Lo and behold, he was admitted a few weeks ago. I didn't go in to see him right away, and when I did, he turned around and he said, "Oh, there you are. I wondered when you'd come in. I would like to know if you would like to work for me." He was an executive with an AIDS research organization, and he said, "You have the most amazing ability to get a group to work together and be just as nice and supportive as you are. How do you do that?" I was almost thrown back out of the room. I said, "What? I didn't even think you'd remember me." He said, "Of course I remember you," and every time someone would walk into the room, he'd say I was wonderful.

Nurses' families surprise them too. Several nurses said that their own families had become active in HIV education and volunteer efforts for AIDS programs. Toby B. went on to say:

> My mother and father have always been proud of me, but now my mother's done AIDS education to her office staff. It's a "my daughter

says" type of thing. My father also. But the one I was most surprised about was my brother. I was just amazed at how much my brother talked about what I did. I always thought he didn't. He never said he wasn't proud of me or anything, but now I meet people he works with and they say, "Oh, you're the one who works in the AIDS unit. Your brother's told me about you."

There has been a change in the past year or so, according to some of the nurses I interviewed, in the public's perception of health-care workers who are involved in HIV care. Whereas earlier nearly everyone connected with the disease, whether patient or caregiver, was avoided and derided, now the feeling is frequently that those who choose to do this work are admirable. This naturally supports these nurses' own image of what they are doing. As Agnes S. said, "I am adventurous, I am courageous. I am a pioneer." By tackling the unfamiliar, nurses discover new capacities within themselves.

For some nurses the route to HIV nursing itself was through self-discovery, a self-discovery fostered by a maturing understanding of what nursing is or can be. As Stephanie C., who has more than twenty years of nursing experience, described the process:

> When I was a young nurse, the thing that I thought was a requisite for job satisfaction was the level of action, what we called the blood and guts. The surgeons, the ICU nurses, they were the most admired. I was a nurse anesthetist for seven years and I loved that. I had a lot of autonomy at the head of the table. It became very technical, more and more instrumentation. The patient was asleep. There was no patient relationship except before and after anesthesia, so I found that what was most satisfying for me was the technical expertise of the job. Then, gradually, as I matured, it got to be routine, repetitious and mechanical. Then my child was diagnosed with a serious disease, and we were exposed to the medical system from the other side, and I saw how important nurses were to the family and to the patient. They really made the difference in the experience of the illness. They didn't change the diagnosis, but it made a difference what nurse was on duty when we went for treatments. There was a particular nurse who was very talented and who really gave of herself, and when she came through the door, my husband and my child and I experienced whatever happened that day in a different way. And that said to me, "Wow, that's what I want to do now," and I went back to school. I went back oriented to new nursing theorists, new ways of looking at nurses and nursing,

> and this became very exciting because I discovered I was very good at it.

Caring for HIV-infected patients can provide a setting within which nurses continue to learn what they do well and how these talents can help the patient. Stephanie C. continued:

> I've learned that I'm very good at conveying the hope in the situation and enabling people to see that each moment is precious, that this moment, living right now, today, is precious. I try to get people to slow down time, to enjoy each other, to go for a walk. I'm very enthusiastic about life and I think I'm able to convey this. At least patients tell me that that's what they get from me. They get hope from me but a realistic hope.

She went on to say:

> I've learned I'm very good at translating what the doctor said into concrete information that the patient can use, into something that means something to them in their lives. When a doctor comes in and says, "Gee, your numbers look good, we'll discharge you tomorrow," the patient needs to know what that means. What I do is tell the family, "She's going home tomorrow but she's going to be very weak. She'll slowly need building up and you do that by good food, lots of rest, let her listen to music or whatever she likes to do." And then I ask the patient, "What do you like to do?" and they'll say, "Oh, I like to draw or I like to play with my child or whatever." I enjoy getting engaged with the patient and maintaining that support system for them even after they leave the hospital.

Self-knowledge thus becomes a therapeutic tool. "Knowing who you are," John N. said, "means knowing what you have that can help others. This is what I am and this is what I can do for you." Lipson has described this facet of nursing as "the therapeutic use of the self" (1991: 75).

Using one's "self" in nursing demands an empathic, emotional, and intuitive understanding of the "other," but in practical terms, it also means that the practitioner needs to be skilled at "observing how one's own behavior and feeling affect clients and being aware of one's own style of interaction, values, and attitudes" (Lipson 1991: 75). At the same time, one must tailor one's own actions to the style of the "other," to his or her values and attitudes. This means, for example, being able to give bad news without devastating the patient or family. As Stephanie C. describes it:

> If you explain to people what the doctors don't have time to do, or maybe they don't have the skills to do, the patients are very grateful. They will say, "Oh, thank you, nobody ever explained that before," or, "That medication, I didn't know it would do that to my son." It's very hard, for example, for the family to learn that the patient is going to lose mental capacities, that he might be sitting, drooling in a chair before long, so they'd better be prepared. It should be done in the kindest way. There are ways of telling people without chopping off their feet. You can leave them with crutches.

Thus, the "other" must always be taken into account. The nurse learns to consider how her or his words are received and the implications they have for others. Sometimes the nurse learns not to ask questions, learns to leave well enough alone, learns that what she or he thought of as a simple query can cause profound pain. The nurse learns that what looks simple can be very complex. As one participant said:

> The latest trend [in families] is that the young mother's often out on the street on drugs and the maternal grandmother steps into the picture. This is a woman who is older, and she now has all these small children to raise. I remember one particular grandmother, the child was in the hospital constantly, and the grandmother and her husband were just exhausted. And I said to her, "Where's the mother [of this child]?" And she looked out the window, and she said, "She's out there somewhere." And the look on her face, this wistful look, I learned not to ask that question. I just say now, "And the child's mother is?" and let her finish it however she wants to. I keep it contained. I don't ask open-ended questions anymore. I use close-ended questions to spare them the pain.

Part of learning about oneself includes learning what one cannot do. This is valuable information too and can promote collaboration and collegiality with other members of the health-care team. Nurses of HIV-infected patients have to work within the framework of their own and their patients' capabilities and they have to accept both their own and their patients' limitations. Stephanie C. said of herself:

> There are some patients I've learned I can't deal with very well and some others can. That's why one's coworkers are so important. For

> example, ——— is much less judgmental than I am. He's very important to me because I know I can always go to him and say, "I'm having trouble with this patient," and he'll help out. I have trouble with substance abusers and alcoholics. Up to a point, I'm able to work with them. In general, I'm able to work with them. My trouble starts when I see people using drugs and beating their children, beating their wives or husbands, not keeping their clinic appointments, and then coming back and being very demanding, and insisting on getting seen ahead of other patients. I have a lot of trouble with that. I feel that we're working so hard and doing such a good job here, and when these people come in, and they use the most terrible language, very abusive language, and they come right into the clinic and say, "I know I missed my clinic appointment three months ago, but I have to be seen right now because I'm sick." And you look at them, and you see the fresh tracks on their arms, and you know they've been stealing and shooting up. At that point, I get impatient. ——— never does. And I know that when I feel this coming, all I have to do is drop back to the second line; ——— takes over. I can do the same thing for him. You learn where you need support and how and where to find it. I've learned my limitations.

In this process of recognition, reflection, and response between themselves and their patients, the nurses I interviewed become clearer to themselves and to others. In this way, attitudes and assumptions are revealed. Customary ways of thinking and behaving are examined. What was perhaps only known to themselves, or known as a latent power or attribute, becomes visible to all. As Watts and Williams remark, "It is a psychological truism that self awareness and self realisation are achieved in the context of personal relationships" (1988: 103). It may even be that self-awareness and self-realization are not possible outside relations with others. As Malson says: "Before his encounter with others, man is nothing but a notional quantity as thin and insubstantial as mist. To acquire his substance, he requires a milieu—the presence of others" (1972: 10).

Nursing almost always includes personal relationships. It therefore offers its practitioners a venue conducive to self-actualization. In others' reaction to them, the nurses in this study frequently find the approval that supports their desire to act in ways consistent with their principles. Through their patients' responses, in what families say, in what doctors do, these nurses see themselves as others see them, and what they see pleases them. They see people who are intelligent and knowledgeable, people who are strong, people who are active, people who are virtuous. Who they are develops through their involvement in

HIV nursing. This is dynamic learning. As the disease changes and as the patients change, nurses learn new things about the disease, about patients, and about themselves.

HIV care is thus not for those who are unsure of themselves, who have doubts about what they are or might be, who need to buttress their sense of self with denial or fantasy. In order to be open to others, a practitioner must be self-aware and self-accepting, so that the deficiencies of other people become a bond rather than a barrier. Those who are open to what people at the margins can teach them will be attracted to caring for HIV-infected patients because learning about others is a form of learning about oneself. If this contact is entered into openly and freely, the occasion of contact "has the ability to expand human capacities" (Watson 1988: 59).

HIV-infected patients bring into the hospital or the clinic all the social problems of the inner city. They are the homeless, the disconnected, the marginal. Their lives and their needs are very different from their middle-class caregivers, but in that difference can lie opportunities for discovery. As Stephanie C. said:

> I have a patient now who is a bilateral amputee. He has KS of both feet and legs and he had to have both his legs amputated. He's a young black man who's been in the hospital for months; he's now in the rehab unit. He's homeless; he has a sister but she refuses to take him. He asked me about ——— Hospital [a long-term care facility] because they wanted to place him there. He was adamantly refusing to go, but he did ask me, and I said to him, "Several years ago, I went there with a nursing school class to visit, and I was very impressed. They have parks there, and sidewalks, and everything is arranged so that patients can go about by themselves." I told him I saw patients going out to get pizza by themselves. I was very impressed by what I saw. So I told him and I explained what the rooms were like; it was like a dormitory. I said that each patient had posters on the wall and his eyes lit up, and he said, "I could have my own corner?" And I said, "Yes, your own corner and your own bed, and you could put pictures on the wall. You could even start picking out the pictures now that you want to bring." Well, he wheeled himself down the hall and he started to say, "You know what she said, she said I could go to ——— and I'm on the list already; I'm waiting for a bed." This tore me up. All he wants is a little corner, a nook, a little bit of sunshine. I said to myself, "This is a great thing to do, to be able to pick up on this." Sometimes our ideas of patients' needs are grandiose. I keep forgetting to be more concrete, less abstract. It's the same lesson I have to learn over and over again. It's the small things that matter.

In this encounter, the nurse finds that her standards of space and privacy differ from her patient's but, because of her empathic understanding of his response, she is made aware of and participates in his feeling of joy. She does not duplicate his feeling but, through empathy, allows it to resonate within her own being. In so doing, she is awakened to possibilities that lie outside her own experience. As one nursing theorist describes this process: "The call and response of an authentic dialogue between a nurse and a patient has great power—the power to change the lived experience of both patient and nurse— . . . she becomes more than she was before the dialogue" (Paterson and Zderad 1988: iv).

Becoming more depends on the nurse's ability to learn from patients. That in turn hinges on the nurse's understanding that her own experience is not the sum total of possible human behavior. Remaining open to "possibility" enables the nurse to extend her conception of what it means to be human.

Chapter 8
Nursing Consciousness and the Cycle of Life and Death

The knowledge the nurses in this study develop about themselves and their patients is achieved through human relationships, and as such, it is a kind of knowledge disdained by the prevailing ideology of the American medical system. The American medical system is founded on physical science and on the use of the scientific method. It relies on empirically demonstrable effects, and it fosters an "objective" stance. American medicine relies on the belief that each disease has a known etiology and a natural history that plays itself out the same way in each individual patient. Treatment is therefore the same for every patient. The goal is to control and eliminate the source of the disease using drugs and/or surgery (Payer 1988; Starr 1982).

Nursing seeks rather to mobilize the patient's own resources in response to disease. Part of that mobilization will be aided by medical interventions, but only part. Mobilization will also depend on the nurse's ability to elicit and sustain health-enhancing behavior from the patient. Nurses seek to understand and use what they know to foster a process that occurs within the patient. It is not imposed from outside. Thus nurses think along with patients rather than for them. They listen; they believe. As Marcia B. said about "difficult" IVDU patients:

> I think it usually boils down to if the patient tells you something, you can't discount what they're saying to you. The drug abuser, the AIDS patient who is going crazy, they're not just screaming because of their personality; it's their underlying need that perhaps led them to use drugs in the first place.

Nurses, without being made fools of, have to believe their patients. They are skeptical at the patient's peril.

Nursing operates within a web of relationships and succeeds through the efficacy of these relationships. This is why, when medicine has nothing more to offer, there is still a great deal for nursing to do. Some would even say that nursing continues after death, as the nurse tends to the last duties to the body (Wolf 1988).

It is to the patient's body and through the patient's body that the nurse promotes healing, and it is through ministration to the body that a nurse's consciousness is developed. It is a consciousness embedded in and drawing strength from natural life. It does not seek to control and direct natural phenomena through force; it seeks to influence natural phenomena through collaboration and persuasion.

For nurses, the natural world can help, because nursing accepts humanity's animality. American culture, with its well-known insistence on personal cleanliness, strives to forget that human beings produce fluids and products as an accompaniment to life (Perin 1988). But nurses learn to overcome their repugnance to bodily fluids, a repugnance ingrained in American society and eminently expressed in the stigma attached to HIV disease. Part of nurses' training is to accept the byproducts of human life. As one nurse said about coming to terms with HIV disease: "Anyone caring for the sick or injured must overcome their recoil from body fluids at the outset. . . . This disease has brought back all the fears and distastes we had to learn to control in nursing school."

Nursing accepts the conditions of human life: that people have bodies; that human life is experienced within bodies; that bodies, with attendant pleasures and pains, are a part of every human experience. Because human beings have bodies, they cannot escape the imperatives of organic existence, the fact that life is a continuum from birth to death. This is a progression no one evades. Thus all human beings are engaged in a recurring drama in which individuals are born, they live, and then they die. But others will take their place. And so the cycle never ends. Through this cycle all human beings are linked to their fellows, both those past and those to come, so that the past and the future are incorporated into the present. Eliade (1954) calls this "the continuous present" or "mythical time" in which the here and now is inseparable from the past and the future, and what has happened before will happen again.

A recurring cycle of birth and death is the reality of human life, a backdrop against which individuals play out their lives. Recognizing this reality enables nurses to accept the inevitabilities inherent in human life and to accept them as inescapable conditions. They do not try to avoid these conditions; they see them as the mark of humanity. This is what it means to be a human being, subject to pain and decline. As Roberta M., who worked in a world-renowned teaching hospital, said:

> Nobody goes through life completely free of pain, sorrow, hurt, or any of the horrible feelings. Everybody in their life experiences some horrible, painful situations. I think that this has been reaffirmed since I worked on this unit because I see such horrible, horrible things that nobody deserves. Nobody should suffer like these people do.

In this conception of life, pain and sorrow know no boundaries. They come to all. Everyone, at some point in their lives, will be vulnerable, unable to care for themselves, and dependent on others. This is an understanding central to these nurses' consciousness of human life. It underlies Alice D.'s decision to teach. She said: "Someday I'm going to be sick, and I want a competent, caring person taking care of me, and that's one of the reasons I'm in teaching. I want to educate the next generation for the next generation who are going to be sick."

Rich and poor, black and white, men and women, everyone who lives will know what suffering is. As Roberta M. said:

> We all have our issues, including the people who are so-called privileged. They may have problems that may not be financial but are very painful. For example, gay men who have lived in the closet who now have to come out and tell their parents, or perhaps they have to talk to their parents and tell them for the first time that they are gay and that they have AIDS. Or they've had multiple deaths among their friends—all their friends are dying or have died—or there might be two lovers who both have AIDS, one is going, the other one is helping out and knows that he will go eventually, too. That's devastating.

It is this understanding that we all suffer because we are all human that draws the nurse to the patient and which defines the "patient" as a human being in need of care. This understanding is expressed in the gestures of human concern that are the hallmarks of the practice of nursing: the outstretched hand, the physical contact, the solace and comfort given through the body. As Nora J. said:

> No matter how big and strong you are, how many muscles you have, you still have to worry about how your family is going to accept this. Are you going to lose your significant other? Are you going to lose your friends? Every HIV-infected patient asks at one time or another, "Am I going to be alone? Am I going to be an outcast? Who is going to take care of me?" No matter what walk of life they come from, they are all going through the same thing.

Accepting the inevitabilities of human life may be part of these nurses' personal growth and development, but it is not easy. As Roberta M. said about a dying patient:

> I don't deal with it so well. I try to work as hard as I can, that's really what I'm doing, but I often feel very sad. For example, I have one woman here now, she was just admitted, but I had seen her in clinic. One of the physicians referred her to me. She's end-stage. She's in a wheelchair. She's blind. She has a child who has AIDS. She came in yesterday and I hardly recognized her. And this morning at eight o'clock, I ran into her room to see her. I'm obsessed with her. I'm not denying that; I just go and see how she's doing and get tearful and feel awful that this is the end. I wish I could say that I don't, that I had these wonderful coping mechanisms in place. No, no, it's terrible, it's terrible.

When nurses accept inevitability, they accept pain and grief and terror. But they also discover a source of community within that acceptance and so they create a defense against the pain and terror. Against the background of death and sorrow, the practice of the nurses I interviewed establishes that there are other certainties that can be sustained by human beings. Human beings live and die, for that there is no choice, but the manner of their living and dying can be chosen. Nursing practice, for these nurses, becomes a continual enactment and reenactment of this truth.

The practice these nurses espouse combines two views of human beings: first, that each individual plays out a story common to all and, second, that each individual can affect how that story is experienced. Each individual is important and her or his particular history has meaning; at the same time, there is an eternal flow of life, expressed as the journey from birth to death, in which all men and women participate no matter what their individual experiences. For the human race, what is ultimately important is the cycle of birth and death, but recognition of this universal truth results not in a nihilistic rejection of life but in a realization of its worth and value for the individual.

For the nurses I interviewed, the preciousness of human life is expressed in the care they give their patients. In a world where much is unstable and where values shift, nursing affirms that people should be protected and that the fullest experience of living is found in caring relationships with other human beings. These nurses' insistence on taking care of the whole person is an insistence that life is a unitary experience, that we feel with our bodies and our minds, that we think with our bodies and our feelings, that we act with our minds and our feelings. Human experience is all of these things together (Barrett 1990). This perspective enables nurses to respond to more than clinical signs and symptoms.

Thus what the nurses in this study find in their profession is an opportunity to experience the unity of what Western culture has separated for analytic purposes into separate categories: the sensory realm, the rational, and the emotional. As Jacques Maquet says: "Intellectuality and affectivity, volition and action are easily distinguishable concepts in our ordinary communication" (1986: 166). In nursing, however, the subjective and objective are used together. Feelings, thought, and action are intertwined. As Stephanie C. said, "It's not a case of either/or. We have to have both [objective and subjective understanding]."

In caring for the sick, the nurses I interviewed experience and create an encounter that exemplifies these concepts. Their work becomes an expression of these truths. Each episode with a patient is an opportunity to make these values real. All of a nurse's faculties are needed. An active intelligence and disciplined emotions are brought to bear on sensory experience. In contact with a patient, these nurses can establish a relationship in which collaboration is more important than control, where self-assertion is restrained, but in which selfhood—the selfhood of both the nurse and the patient—can be experienced fully. One nurse commented: "It's a privilege to be there." As Watson says of such encounters: "The nurse is able to form a union with the other person on a level that transcends the physical . . . [but] preserves the subjectivity and physicality of persons. . . . There is a freeing of both persons from their separation and isolation" (1988: 68).

This kind of experience does not occur in every nursing encounter and nurses do not expect that it will. But nurses can frame the relationship. The nurse is in charge; she (or he) can resist being drawn into the patient's perspective and can refuse or cut short an episode that is not going well. The nurse can come back later and try again, when the patient seems more amenable. In this way, a nurse can maintain independence at the same time that she or he remains open and accessible to the patient. Thus, even in the most beleaguered situations, there is always the possibility of an encounter in which patient and nurse agree to act together, recognizing and respecting each other's humanity. As one nurse said of the patient-caregiver relationship:

> It's a connectedness within which there's trust, there's freedom to be who you are. It's non-judgmental. Particularly when I'm working with prisoners, they tell me things that make the hair on the back of my Anglo-Saxon neck stand straight up, but at the same time I can

> see that these prisoners, for whatever reason they got into this predicament, they need a nurse. And I'm there, and I can be there for them. They need an advocate. And I can maintain their dignity in a situation which could be demeaning. HIV patients have to tell me all sorts of details which ordinarily no one else would ever know. I try to make it as easy as possible for them, while still getting the information I need. I give them the tools they need to build their lives again. They come in. They are at the bottom. And then I tell them how they can help themselves. I want to give them some sort of string to hold on to, even if it's the tiniest thread. You have to give them something to hold onto, even if it's just for a day, or an hour. Just to let them know that you care. We may not understand what they're going through, but we can let them know we care.

When nursing is conducted in this fashion, it is as though many of the walls, psychic and social, preventing contact between individuals are breached or erased. The constraints of ordinary human life disappear and a freer, more generous mode of human interaction becomes possible. This is experienced as freedom. It is a freedom to establish a relationship with another human being unrestrained by worldly considerations or by functional rationality. In such a relationship, these nurses find the freedom to be themselves while caring for their patients. As Chris T. said about caring for IV drug users:

> If you're decent to them, they're very, very grateful, and you can interact in a way that's a little freer. I don't know how to describe it exactly. They're a tough group and they don't tolerate any bullshit. You can't run anything by them. But, on the other hand, you can be very frank with them, and they appreciate some of that stuff that other people might find offensive or something. I don't know how to describe it exactly. You have to work with a different attitude about your goals and your aims and your measure of success.

The freedom found in caring for HIV-infected patients comes from a paradoxical acceptance of limitation. It is an acceptance of the human condition, that there is good and bad, hope and despair, laughter and tears. Human life is composed of a host of opposites: courage and cowardice, kindness and contempt, loyalty and betrayal. As Hubert Benoit states, "In refusing to accept limitations, man deprives himself of the impression of liberty which he feels when he is within accepted constraints" (1955: 66). The nurses I interviewed accept the limitations inherent in human life. This enables them to focus on that which is not finite, the capacity to connect with other human beings.

Chapter 9
Nursing as a Moral Undertaking

As documented in the American Nurses' Association Code of Ethics, nurses are not allowed to pick and choose their patients. They must care for the patients assigned to them. Anyone who is ill is worthy of attention, and that attention should be the same whether the sick person is poor or rich, black or white, female or male; social categories should not matter. Whoever comes to the unit, or registers for home care, or signs up at the clinic is to be treated, and to be treated to the same standards. As Alice D. explained:

> The National League for Nursing has come out with guidelines that say that this [learning about AIDS] should be part of nursing education. Because now you just can't say, "Well, I won't work on an AIDS unit," because AIDS patients are going to be all over. They're everywhere and you're not going to be able to refuse, even if it were ethically correct, which it is not. Nurses are going to have to come to grips with this. It's slow going but it's coming. Nurses are doing better than doctors. Maybe it's because we're not given as much choice. We're not private practitioners. Doctors can, regardless of their pronouncements, they can pick and choose. They can just say, "I'm not really qualified to take care of AIDS patients. You're really better off going to a doctor who is an AIDS specialist." They have an out. Nurses don't have that out.

In caring for HIV-infected patients, the nurses in this study were honoring the moral principles of their profession. Behind the focus and interest on clinical issues, which are foremost in nurses' own discussions of the disease, there lies a code of ethics which directs and informs practice. This ANA code has been clearly articulated in the statements of the Association of Nurses in AIDS Care, a professional organization dedicated to the promotion of the health and welfare of people infected with HIV disease. The Association's statement on nurses' duty to care says that "all professional nurses have a responsibility to deliver care to HIV-infected individuals regardless of risk factor, lifestyle, racial or ethnic group" (*Journal of the Association of Nurses in AIDS Care* 1991: 44).

The nurses I interviewed believe in this code and they practice with this code in mind. They are committed professionals whose nursing practice is more than a technical task. In caring for HIV-infected patients, they are making a moral statement. None of the nurses I interviewed believed that nurses should be able to pick and choose their patients. Such a stance does not mean that these nurses would force workers to care for HIV-infected patients, but it does mean that a hospital nurse or a home-care nurse must accept whichever patients are on their roster. As Robin M. said:

> You cannot choose. I don't think you can. I don't know exactly how medicine or surgery work, but I know, for nurses, you cannot refuse an assignment. And how do I feel about it? I think it's wonderful. Of course if you choose to work in AIDs, you don't take risks, and you're very very careful. But I don't think that any one of us should refuse to take care of anyone, even if you don't agree with the person's lifestyle. That is not the point.

In choosing HIV care, these nurses are putting their bodies, their minds, and their hearts behind their beliefs. They are acting according to the highest ideals of nursing. And they are acting freely; they all have had opportunities, because of their education and experience, to take positions that would not bring them into such constant contact with HIV disease.

Because other health professionals they come in contact with do not always agree with them, these nurses not infrequently find themselves at odds with workers operating from a different moral framework. As Alison J., who worked in a municipal hospital, said:

> It's a real problem, like finding a patient in full distress, and the doctor hasn't been up there in a few days, and you know he's not coming. We had a patient who left our unit, but had to stay in the hospital because he didn't have a place to go, so they put him on the service where they're supposed to be given supportive care, and he had to come back to us because he became acutely ill. This is someone who was in a hospital! He was under the care of a physician. He became dehydrated. That should never happen in a hospital. He also had thrush, it was all up his nose; he looked like a rabid dog, his

> thrush was so bad. That was obscene as far as I'm concerned. I blame the nursing staff almost as much as the doctors. I have never seen thrush like that. He couldn't open his mouth. And it's so easily treated. There's a wafer, and if that doesn't work, there's a liquid, like a swish and swallow. Sometimes that doesn't work and you need a systemic, which we gave this man, and within a week, he was okay. But, as I say, nobody listens to me.

Because of the hierarchy within the American medical system, and because of the traditional relationship between nurses and doctors in this system, nurses often have to be extremely persistent in order to get HIV-infected patients the proper care, particularly in municipal hospitals. Alison J. went on to say:

> I have walked into rooms and found patients seizing, and they haven't drawn bloods for two or three weeks. Then, if you want to go to a specialist, if there's a special problem, we've just been told recently to stop doing that, to go instead to the primary physician and ask him to call in the specialist, like a neurologist. Most of the time the primary physician just tells us, "Yeah, yeah, yeah," and they don't take any action.

In the face of such reactions, it is hard not to give up, but these nurses don't. They make the calls. They keep after physicians. Alison J. described how she pursued one patient's doctor: "I don't pretend to be able to diagnose everything, but some things are very obvious. For one patient, I called the doctor to say the potassium was really high. She said, 'Oh?' so I told her, 'Why don't you do this, this and this'; 'Oh, okay,' she said. But three days later I went back, and she hadn't looked at the results, so I had to call her again." Another nurse said, somewhat wistfully, "It's a battle. If you're not really assertive, you're not going to survive." Another commented that she always seemed to have more energy to keep pushing for the patients on Mondays; by Friday, she was less apt to keep after things.

Some nurses find it hard to maintain their own hope and optimism in the face of their patients' experiences. It is a struggle to accept the limitations of what can be done. As Gretchen S. said: "[At the beginning] I would want to do more and more and more, and I think just the realization that you can't do more took a while. Not that you shouldn't try, but at some point, there are going to be many people for whom you can't do more." Actually just getting what can be done done is hard work. Many of the nurses I interviewed said that persisting in the face of difficulties and failure was something they had to work at. Gretchen S. explained what she regularly came up against in a municipal hospital:

> Take, for example, the CAT scan. They [the patients] have two choices. They can go to the emergency room, and they can wait in line to get a bed, which would take two or three days, so they can get a CAT scan. Or they could try to go over and get an emergency CAT scan which would probably take six weeks. Now I can spend a lot of energy trying to manipulate this, making calls, going here, going there. But I can't get you a CAT scan appointment as an outpatient. They're not going to give it to you. Nobody's going to give it to you no matter how you carry on.

The inequities and inadequacies of the New York City health-care system have been made very obvious by HIV disease. One nurse who directed a foster care agency for AIDS pediatric patients in one of New York's outer boroughs said: "After two years, we were finally able to locate a dentist willing to care for HIV children, but for a good neurological workup we still have to come into Manhattan. We're just now [1991] starting aerosol pentamidine. This disease has magnified the failures of the health-care system." These failures existed before HIV disease and will exist after, but even for nurses in voluntary and not-for-profit hospitals, there is a belief that the HIV-infected patient is not a top priority. Medicaid patients everywhere do not get the latest treatment. And in the municipal system, as one nurse put it, "The administration would be happy if they [the HIV-infected patients] would all just hurry up and die."

In a situation where assumptions and goals are contested, nurses have to be very clear about their own position. Chris T. told this story:

> We had a doctor who cut himself while performing a minor operation of a seventy-plus patient. He nicked himself and he felt exposed. And he came in and he said to me, "I want you to test her [for HIV]." And I said, "You have to sign that form." And he said, "I want you to send her blood for testing." And I said, "You have to sign that form." The confidentiality law had just been passed which requires informed consent from the patient. He said, "I shouldn't have to get her permission. I just need to know. I shouldn't have to get her permission." I said, "I won't send her blood." He said, "You have to send her blood. I'm telling you to send her blood." I said, "I will not send her blood." I said, "You do not have a signed consent form. You do whatever you want, but I will not send the blood without a signed

> consent form." I said even if it wasn't illegal, which it was, it was unethical. So I would not do it. What I think he was trying to do was get me to do what he wanted to do, so that he would have an accomplice, so that it would make what he wanted to do right in some way. I said, "Here are the forms, you fudge them, you're a doctor, you can lie about this stuff, you go ahead and do it and send it, but I won't do it for you. I'm telling you how to do it and break the law; you go ahead and do it."

Nurses have to be strong to do this work. They must be able to control their emotions. They must be able to withstand the opprobrium attached to caring for people with HIV disease. They have to deal with their own fears and ambivalent feelings. They have to manage many patients who find it difficult to be compliant. They have to maintain a positive outlook despite the fact that treatments merely delay the inevitable. They have to manipulate the bureaucracy and, in many cases, challenge the power of doctors. They have to contend with a fragmented and crisis-ridden medical system. None of these conditions is exclusive to HIV infection, but HIV disease exacerbates them. As Emma B. described it:

> I used to come home feeling that somebody had placed bricks on my shoulders, metaphorically and really, and not just the health issues but the philosophical issues. You get hit in the face with inadequate health care every day, you know that Medicaid patients are not getting the same care as the people with private insurance, you just know it, and you know that a lot of your patients don't want to go to the hospital because they're going to end up on the wards where it's absolute hell. There's a fragmentation issue too, when somebody has Medicaid, and they shuffle from clinic to clinic. If you have three or four diseases, you go to three or four clinics, none of whom are talking to each other, and they all lose your records anyway every time you're there. The paperwork during the Reagan administration tripled, because everything had to be justified, and also they are deliberately making you write more, to slow you down, also to discourage you from providing service to begin with.

Some nurses in the study defined what they did as simply what they were trained in nursing school to do. As Marcia B. said:

> I was taught from day one, "You are the patient's advocate, you have to take care of all these needs." We spent a lot of time learning how to communicate with people, studying the social sciences, and a lot of

other things which weren't strictly nursing. We were taught to look at emotional needs.

This is the holistic nursing ideal, and it is indeed something that nurses have to embrace if they are to be effective with HIV-infected patients. But there must be something more. Nurses have to demonstrate in their practice a belief in the merit and worth of the individual, no matter what that individual is like, no matter what he or she has done. Nora J. put it succinctly:

> In the prison unit, I've taken care of people who were rapists, who were murderers, and my philosophy always has been that you leave your political convictions outside the door. You have to leave what you feel about certain classes of people outside the door. This is a patient. Especially with the prisoners, I used to say, this is a patient who is a prisoner who is a person.

And as Paula T. said about her IV drug users:

> I like them. They're difficult but they're very good. Underneath all that other stuff that people make judgments about, they're really good people who just have had a bad break, or have had society's own judgment about the way people act or their sexual preference. I don't agree with that. I just feel that they're victims.

In this world every person has value. He or she may have almost no social value, but they always retain moral value. It is this moral value which these nurses honor and which they sustain through their practice. As they care for IV drug users and gay men, for women unlucky to have loved infected men, for men unlucky to have loved infected women, for hemophiliacs, for children who will not live long, they are making a statement. What they are saying is that human life is, no matter how short, no matter how abused, no matter how squalid, of great worth.

This is why the issues of the DNR order and pain control are so important to many of the nurses I interviewed. Talking about death and dying, presenting a piece of paper to a patient and watching him or her sign, helping a patient think about what is going to happen, all of these things are not easy. But if they are not done, if these issues are not explored, the patient may not die with dignity. Dying in pain, stripped of the chance to choose, is not a human death. For more than one nurse I interviewed, making sure that patients die well has become the reason for staying with HIV care. This is the ultimate recognition of the patient's humanity, of the bond between the nurse and the patient. It is a declaration of the nurse's humanity as well. As one nursing theorist has said: "If the nurse doesn't recognize the humanity of the patient, the patient is not the only one reduced to an object. The nurse is as well" (Watson 1988: 60). And thus the images of nursing that these nurses retain are images of human connection. Gretchen S. said: "I like thinking about nursing as walking with a patient arm in arm. That's sort of my picture. I might be a little stronger, but it's side by side. And maybe she leans on me, but there's something reciprocal there." Most nurses picture themselves sitting by or on their patients' beds, holding their hand. Most said that when they thought of themselves as a nurse they pictured themselves listening to a patient, or saw themselves talking with a patient, or giving physical care. The model most of us have of this kind of interaction is that of mothers and children, so it is not surprising that many nurses compared what they did to what mothers do. One male nurse said: "It's funny, really, I'm a man, but I picture nursing as someone in a white uniform, a woman bending over a bed, soft lights, the whole works." Nina H. said:

> Nurses are nurturing, think of the word "nursing," the whole meaning, where it comes from, which came first. I think the whole idea of nursing came from taking care of infants. It's like mothering. Not that you're not still doing dressings, and doing IVs and handling suctioning and nine million other nursing functions, but the feeling is you're sort of mothering them, showing concern, showing you care.

It is striking that the images most of these nurses, even those who are men, have of themselves as nurses are those frequently associated with maternal responsibilities and actions: listening, talking, giving physical care. Perhaps that is because maternal care is the best model we have, as a society, of disinterested concern for another human being. Perhaps also it is through such care that a "sense that the world and body are trustworthy and capable" can be restored (Benner 1989: 163).

Maternal care is also the vehicle for a message about life itself. As Peter Berger says:

> The role that a parent takes on represents not only the order of this or that society, but order as such, the underlying order of the universe that it makes sense to trust. It is this role that may be called the role of high priestess. It is a role that the mother in this scene [reassuring a child after a nightmare] plays willy-nilly, regardless of her own awareness or (more likely) lack of awareness of just what it is

> she is representing. "*Everything* is in order, *everything* is all right"—this is the basic formula of maternal and paternal reassurance. Not just this particular anxiety, not just this particular pain, but everything is all right. The formula can, without in any way violating it, be translated into a statement of cosmic scope—"Have trust in being." (1990a: 62; italics in original)

If this is in some part the message of nursing, it is not surprising that it is transmitted in images of an attentive woman, and why, even for men, the practice of nursing can be visualized in female terms.

It has become something of a cliché in the literature on nursing and HIV disease to say that AIDS has brought about a return to valuing "caring" (Fox, Aiken, and Messikomer 1990). Caring is seen as the emotional component of care, but many of the nurses I interviewed were careful to point out that good care does not necessitate emotional involvement. They made a distinction between caring for and caring about. Martha C. said:

> Any nurse is able to care *for* a patient, but I think to care *about* a patient allows you to invest a little bit more. It is not a prerequisite though, you don't have to love all the people you care for. But you do have to see if it's interfering. Is it just that you don't spend much time with them? Or is it that you're holding back pain medicine because they're obnoxious? Or you don't clean them up because they're obnoxious, you make them wait? No, you don't do that, but if you don't take the extra time to sit down with them, it can affect the care. You have to think about it. You have to say to yourself, "Why am I not doing this? Is it better for the patient not to, or is it just that I don't want to go in and bother with him?"

Because nursing is a moral statement, its practitioners must be aware of their own actions, reactions, and motivations. They have to be self-aware and self-correcting. Nurses have to continually question their actions and reactions. They cannot simply follow their inclinations. Emma J. added this comment:

> I just think that to be a good nurse you don't have to love these people. You have to really like people, you can't be just technically correct or you're missing something, and so is the patient. It makes such a difference if the patient feels you really care. You can do that without "caring," because you're going to meet patients you don't like. We have discussions about this [on the unit] all the time.

There are always some patients who forge real affective bonds with nurses. Every nurse I interviewed had favorite patients, patients they would never forget, but the fact that good care is given even when the patients are not liked is the clearest proof that the nursing described by the participants in this study is a moral act. It is done because it is the right thing to do. It is the right thing to do because this is how people should be treated. Thus, for these nurses, what they are doing is the expression of a social vision in which all people are equal. Beyond race, beyond class, beyond gender, beyond any kind of social criteria, the patient, as patient, is entitled to decent care. As Maria J. said:

> I can't imagine being in these patients' position, but I feel that if I was, I would hope that there was someone who was treating me sensitively, would really sit down and talk to me, who I could feel comfortable enough with so I could open up to that person, and that that person would be sensitive and have a lot of knowledge about the disease, would know what I was feeling, the pain, the side effects of medication. I would want someone like that to be available to me.

For the nurses I interviewed the goal is to be that kind of nurse, a nurse who can find a way to communicate with, care for, and comfort any kind of patient. For such a nurse, the connection with the patient becomes the avenue by which moral values and concepts are confirmed and celebrated.

In this sense, nursing is not just about patient care; it is about something else as well. It is the elaboration of a moral order in which people as people, pure and simple, take the foremost place, and in which, as a result, the protection and care of people becomes the most important goal.

Chapter 10

Death and Transcendence

There are several reasons why a moral vision that holds people to be of the highest value is critical to caring for HIV-infected patients. The first reason is that the disease is prevalent among groups on the margins of society. It was in the homosexual communities in both New York and San Francisco that the disease first became manifest. Although these communities were active and visible, they were also isolated from mainstream society. Unless nurses worked within these communities, they would not normally meet these patients in their work.

IV drug users were even less likely to have much contact with health-care personnel, except in drug treatment programs or in emergency care settings. Thus, the sudden appearance of large numbers of gay patients and IV drug users in health-care settings in the 1980s was a shock to many nurses. Even if they worked in municipal hospitals, nurses had never had so many gay men or substance abusers as patients before HIV disease brought them, by the thousands, into the health-care system. Nurses who saw these groups as unworthy of care for some reason, because of moral turpitude or social failure, found it difficult to care for them (Gee 1989). Nurses who saw these patients as people first were more likely to step forward and take care of them.

Furthermore, a moral vision which does not calculate social worth and cost is important because HIV-infected patients require an enormous amount of work but have poor prospects for a positive outcome. They need continual attention, but their response to treatment is always problematical. As Arthur R. described a recent patient:

> I just had a patient who over the course of six weeks [had a succession of crises]. First it was his Hickman [a permanent IV catheter] got infected, then he had new KS [Kaposi's sarcoma] lesions, then he became anemic, and one other thing—I can't remember what—got worse. And it looked as though it was all under control, but actually

> the Hickman infection probably never was under control, so he came into the hospital a couple of weeks ago, and went into shock and almost died. He was in ICU because everything was slightly crazy. They didn't know what was going on because the blood cultures were negative, but something had to be there, something that was not totally killed by the antibiotic. He looked like he was going to die. He was on a respirator, they gave him medication to keep his blood pressure up, he was on three antibiotics, he was unresponsive for a period of time. He was bleeding, and he was pretty much unresponsive, and then, two days later, he got better.

This story could be repeated endlessly. The patient is very ill; everyone works very hard to keep him or her alive. They succeed; the patient lives a little longer but will become ill again in the future, and the sequence of care and partial recovery will be repeated until death.

Although the nurses I interviewed were comfortable with the prospect that, at some point, active treatment should be discontinued, now there is often a long time before patients reach that point, and nurses have to be ready to work hard to keep patients going while their ability to regain a high quality of life declines with each episode of illness. This effort is easiest to maintain when the patient's wishes are considered paramount and when other considerations, such as social and monetary cost and efficiency, are ignored.

This is why all the nurses I interviewed said that decisions about treatment should be left to the patient. They believed that they could provide valuable information to the patient about the consequences of treatment and the cessation of treatment. They also believed that other health professionals had a role to play in informing the patient, so that the patient's decision would be based on sufficient information. If the patient wanted everything done, that was acceptable. If the patient signed a Do Not Resuscitate order and then wanted to rescind it, that was acceptable. If the patient wanted only pain medication, that was also acceptable.

Only one nurse, of all those I interviewed and those who answered the questionnaire, raised the question of cost. For no other nurse was it an issue. The focus was on what patients needed and how it could be provided. At least with me, there was no discussion of how to allocate resources, or whether resources had to be allocated at all. The assumption was that since HIV-infected patients are people, that was sufficient reason for the effort expended. As Maria J. said: "When nurses get to administration, they don't care about patients. It's just dollars and cents. I never want to be an administrator. I care about patients too much."

This focus on patients and on the moral vision that excludes other considerations is necessary to HIV nursing. And yet it is not sufficient to explain why nurses remain in this kind of nursing and expect to stay with it. It is hard and difficult work with relatively few extrinsic rewards. As Cassie N. said: "Nursing is not pure nursing. There's a little bit of dietary, there's a little bit of being an electrical engineer, there's a little bit of being a doctor, being a janitor, being a handmaiden. It's definitely not what you see on TV."

Yet, despite the demands of nursing—and the nurses I interviewed did not try to gloss over the difficulties they faced—they liked taking care of HIV-infected patients. I believe they liked it because, in caring for HIV-infected patients, they found a way to respond to the central challenge of human life, the inevitability of death. The patients these nurses care for die, but their manner of dying is a statement that death is not the end of life.

One nurse called caring for HIV-infected patients a "gift." It is a gift to both nurse and patient, consisting of the chance to confront death and to construct, nurse and patient together, death's defeat. Accepting this gift brings nurses and patients profound experiences of connection and continuity.

The nurses I interviewed did not speak directly of this aspect of HIV care. They told me that they had to confront their own and their patients' mortality and they expressed a general belief in a continuation beyond death. But they were reticent about how nursing HIV-infected patients enabled them to face death squarely without succumbing to despair. I believe, however, that the practice of nursing as demonstrated by these nurses embodies, literally, the conviction that human beings remain linked through illness, death, and beyond. This conviction underlies all that nurses do. The discussion which follows, therefore, is based on nurses' accounts of what they do, not on how they analyze what they do. It is my interpretation of what, in practice, usually remains unsaid. The fact that it is not said probably contributes to its power.

Nurses and patients first work at keeping death at bay with treatment and care. The success in recent years of treatments for opportunistic infections can make this early stage quite long, but at some point, despite sophisticated medical interventions, death is inevitable. When it becomes clear that death is on the horizon, a transition to another kind of effort emerges. As Stephanie J. said: "There's a transitional period in the middle there where you have to adjust to the fact that the patient is no longer able to maintain their health, and there's a transition period there for both myself and the patient, where we start to prepare for facilitating death and preparing for it."

As death comes closer, the nurse and the patient work together to achieve a sense of the continuity of human life as well as an understanding of the individual's particular place in the cycle of human existence. By affirming the continuity of life, nurse and patient declare death, at this stage, symbolically defeated.

The fact of death is a challenge to every human being's sense of self, because death brings "biological and psychic annihilation" (Lifton 1979: 18). The prospect of death, even for the healthy, often provokes terror and grief, and some people respond to the thought of death by denying both the expectation of death and its meaning. But in most human cultures, the challenge of death has been met differently. Most human societies have sought immortality and have insisted that individual lives are somehow connected to eternity. Part of the horror and poignancy of HIV disease comes from its connection to sex, which is our most direct defense against fears of abandonment and nothingness and our strongest apprehension of immortality, because procreation and reproduction are our most visible links to the future.

A belief in immortality serves as protection against the void, the nothingness, so overwhelming in physical death. It counters the fact of separation with faith in connection. Somehow some element of ourselves lives on, in others' memory or in artifacts left behind. Perhaps the individual's life is incorporated into the divine. For some, intimations of eternity can be apprehended before physical death in transcendental experiences.

The human search for immortality can take several forms. Lifton identifies five responses to death which each incorporate images of eternal time, "a sense of biohistorical continuity" (1979: 18), an endless flow of life. These images are representations of eternity and they offer comfort and balm to human beings struggling with the fact of death. The first and most common approach to immortality is biological, "epitomized by family continuity, living on through—psychologically speaking, *in*—one's sons and daughters and their sons and daughters, with imagery of an endless chain of biological attachment" (Lifton 1979: 18; italics in original). In the family the individual "finds his ancestors continuing mysteriously within himself, and in the same way he projects his own being into his children and later descendents" (Berger 1990b [1967]: 62). Immortality is real because the same life that animated those who went before will animate those who come after. The thinking expressed in this concept is:

> "I must die—but my children and children's children will live on for ever." . . . The entire collectivity, bound together by ties of blood, thus becomes (to its own self-understanding) quite concretely im-

> mortal, for it carries with it through time, the *same* fundamental life which is incarnate in each of its members. (Berger 1990b [1967]: 62; italics in original)

As Lifton points out, this thinking can be easily extended beyond the family to the tribe, the organization, ethnic group, nation, or species. Indeed, for caregivers themselves, it is often important that they feel that their efforts will benefit not only the patient but the patient's family and loved ones. They hope that what they do for the patient carries forward into the lives of the patient's children and onward into the future. Thus, in their service to their patients, practitioners themselves experience this mode of immortality and make it available to their patients.

The second approach to immortality is religious. Through attachment to a particular creed, the believer is "offered the opportunity to be reborn into a timeless realm of ultimate, death-transcending truths" (Lifton 1979: 20). This realm may be a personalized and material one, such as the City of God imagery of the New Testament, or it may be conceived of simply as a flow of divine energy, but essential to any religious vision of the hereafter is a belief in union with God or the divine life force.

Through death, the individual becomes part of the eternal and divine. "For example, the Chinese peasant could die calmly in the assurance that he would live on in his descendents as his ancestors have lived on in him, but the Confucian gentleman could have the same assurance legitimated further by reference to the fundamental *tao* with which his life and his dying were properly attuned" (Berger 1990b [1967]: 63). In this scheme, what happens on earth is incorporated into the divine order. For nurses who believe in life after death, part of their practice, sometimes acknowledged, sometimes not, lies in preparing dying patients for the final step through which individual human lives become part of another more permanent and more perfect world.

A third approach finds immortality in human creativity. Creativity is commonly associated with works of art or science, but it is also a component of other human activities, particularly those which promise permanence. It constitutes monumental architecture's great appeal, some of the drive and energy which infuses business projects, and even the creation of domestic life.

Human action leaves its imprint on the world and on society; thus making a lasting imprint means that one's influence continues after death. For patients, the stories of their lives, the stories they tell their nurses, are ways of saying, "I lived and I did something which lives after me." For nurses themselves, it may be that "making a difference" is one way of achieving immortality.

The fourth approach focuses on man's link to the natural world, "the perception that the natural environment around us, limitless in space and time, will remain" (Lifton 1979: 22) after our deaths. The recurrence of natural rhythms in nature, of death and rebirth, echoes our own pattern. In attuning ourselves to those rhythms, we participate in the limitlessness and eternity of Nature. Our embeddedness in nature becomes, in this mode, an avenue to immortality rather than a proof of our impermanence. Thus nurses' acceptance of the natural world links them to the permanence and infinity of Nature. When individuals are gone, the natural world remains.

The fifth approach to immortality is different in kind from the first four. It is to be found in experiences of transcendence that are characterized by personal feelings of timelessness and infinity. In these instances, the cosmic order itself is felt, and it brings with it a vivid sense of life. Central to such experiences is detachment from immediate concerns and involvements. The self feels permeable, open to outside influences, yet focused and harmonious. As a result, there is "a temporary loss of differentiation of the self and the outer world . . . [that] may lead to a lessening of alienation, to a rediscovery of the self, to a new set of values, to the finding of new potential for growth and development, and to a new beginning" (Lifton 1979: 25).

Both the patient and the nurse, if their encounters reach this level, experience pleasure and joy. They receive intimations of a kind of existence qualitatively different from normal human life, one suffused with ease and satisfaction, contrasting with the anticipation of separation and meaninglessness attached to the prospect of death.

It is my contention that the nurses in this study used all of these various approaches, as situations demanded, in order to reconcile their patients and themselves to the central fact of human existence, the fact that we die. The holistic philosophy of nursing that they espoused enabled them to use many different responses to their patients' needs for reassurance. If they had seen their role as simply clinical, they would not have been able to provide their patients with so many different ways of confronting and overcoming the prospect of death.

A few nurses spoke specifically of their religious commitments and how these helped them in this work. The majority of those I interviewed, however, shied away from religious discussion or interpretation. They were reluctant to consider what they did as religious in any sense, or even spiritual. But labels aside, it seems clear to me that what they were doing was providing a framework within which patients could feel that death was not the absolute end to their lives.

The nurse I spoke with who arranged the photography exhibit for her patient was saying, "Your work lives after you." This was also the message of the video project: Patients would be given the chance to leave a record behind them. They might speak of their love for their children or for their partners and friends. Patients might be filmed at home or at work. One patient was anxious to preserve a record of his concerts. He was a pianist. Just so the memorial services and the quilts and the candles that many nurses use to keep the memory of their patients alive also makes clear to patients that they will not be forgotten.

This is the paradox of caring for HIV-infected patients. The individual patient and the nurse's relationship to that individual are at the center of care, but as the disease progresses, the individuality of the patient, his or her personality, is very likely to disintegrate. The patient declines, physically and mentally, emotionally and psychologically, so that, at the end, the person with whom the nurse has forged a relationship is often gone. This leaves the nurse as witness to the patient as he or she was, not as he or she is at the moment of death. Many nurses in this study recognized that they were being asked to keep memory alive and that this was an important component of nursing. They told me that they talked to the person as they wrapped the body up in the final ritual of care. They described patients' deaths to colleagues who were not present in the last moments. They tried in various ways to keep communal memory alive. As Cassie N. said:

> When we first opened, we did a number of things which we don't do now. Originally we had the idea that we'd take pictures [of patients who had died] and keep a list of who had died when, but then we decided it would be too depressing for the patients still on the unit. We used to hold memorial services once a month on the unit, just with staff who were on duty that day, a memorial to all the patients who had died that month on this unit and on other units. It had a religious overtone but it wasn't any particular religion. We'd read some poetry and we'd list the names, and usually the nurses would break into tears, and then it was over. We'd all go back to work.

As long as people are remembered they are not really gone. One way to preserve memory is to put it into words. Nurses are often asked to listen as patients review their lives. They also sometimes suggest that patients write their stories down, an enterprise that offers permanence and closure. Thus Stephanie C. encouraged one of her patients to start a journal. She said:

> I have a woman upstairs who is doing a journal. She's the editor, she will decide what she wants in it, she's the narrator. She let me read the beginning of her journal, and it said, "Hello, old friend, I received

> you from a lady," and she goes on this way, talking to the journal as if it's a person, a friend whom she can tell anything to. She's a young black woman, thirty or so, and I guess she wanted me to know the pain but not directly, so she recounts [in her journal] an experience where she was raped. She writes like an angel, she could have been a writer. She said, "I'm afraid of this thing called death, I'm afraid it's going to take me like the wind takes the dry leaves and put me out of sight."

By far the most common approach to immortality these nurses used was the biosocial one, the notion that we live on through our connections with other people. If their patients had strong ties to others, these ties had to be maintained. Families, friends, partners, and lovers were welcomed, not excluded. If their patients' connections to others were tenuous or ruptured, they had to be restored—thus the nurses who arranged bedside reconciliations, who fought for custody plans for their patients, who made sure wills were signed, who put dying individuals in touch with their families, friends, partners, and lovers. These patients could feel that something of themselves continued in the world after they themselves were gone. The image of death was replaced with an image of life. The patient could feel "I live on in humankind" (Lifton 1979: 20).

These nurses enable their patients to die well, with a "measure of self-completion" (Lifton 1979: 91), and a sense of integrity. They rescue their patients from disintegration in the face of physical death because their deaths are seen as "part of some immortalizing current of the vast human flow" (Lifton 1979: 91). The individual's experience is connected to a collective "quest for a continuous symbolic relationship to what has gone before and what will continue after our finite individual lives" (Lifton 1979: 17).

This message is conveyed to the patient by the nurse in all the myriad actions of care. These actions can be conceived of as rituals of connection, statements that, though in extremis, the patient will not be abandoned. As Bob G. said of a patient he felt lucky to have visited:

> I remember one day I walked in on a guy I knew, he had a lymphoma of the lung, which is fairly common with AIDS patients. He had pulled out his IV, he was lying with blood all over his bed. He was short of breath, the nebulizer to his oxygen was empty, so he was getting dry oxygen which dries out the mouth. He was just a mess. I put on a gown and gloves and I cleaned him up. I changed the sheets, I got him a blanket, and I got him some ice water for his mouth. Then I filled the nebulizer and put it on to make him a little

> more comfortable. He was dead that afternoon. I know that I had made him comfortable on the day he died, and I said to myself, "Thank God I didn't say, 'Wait until your nurse comes along.'" I just went and did it myself. I've had lots of moments like that.

What these nurses do is affirm their patients' lives as they die. By caring for them, they tell their patients that their lives have meaning, because their death is a part of the larger rhythms of human life. The human condition becomes less frightening, less dreadful. Images of nothingness, of the void of death, are replaced with images of connection. The meaninglessness of death is replaced with the meaning of life, which lies in every human being's participation in the cosmic drama of existence. The individual's insignificance is transformed into significance.

In their practice, the nurses in this study perform actions of connectedness that dispel their own and their patient's fears of rootlessness. They place themselves and their patients in the great chain of being, linking the past to the future. They recover a sense of beginnings and endings and reestablish the "mythical time" (Eliade 1954) within which human life is endlessly renewed.

For the nurse and for the patient, the actions of the nurse represent the link between the patient and all other human beings. The patient becomes the representative of all other individuals who must, at some time, face death. In ministering to the patient, the nurse embodies an image of human connectedness and human continuity. Thus caring for HIV-infected patients becomes a life-affirming act. It is this confirmation of continuity, the sense that one's death is a part of life and that life goes on, which gives the care of HIV-infected individuals its vitality and its power.

The vitality also comes from the fact that it is a relationship with another human being, and that the meaning for the patient is also the meaning for the nurse. The nurse benefits, too. As Gretchen S. said:

> I'm really starting to think about this whole nursing process as an art as well as a science. And it's not something I would have considered before [HIV]. I would have said that if someone were a therapist, they were doing something that was more creative, more skilled, with their patients. I would have said that was not what I do with my patients. I really devalued nursing. But now, a lot because of the intensity of the relationship and the ongoing nature of it, and because there is so much at stake here, I feel there is something very creative, very special going on with people. I'm still working on this and trying to find out what's kind of moving it. But something

> happens, something happens there for me. I can't say for patients, but something happens there for me that is very strong and intense, and real, and also very nourishing for me. I just really feel, and I'm not sure why, I'm just comfortable being there and talking to these people. There's some two-way thing going on. I've just started to think of the value of silence, and just sitting with them, and letting people just know that you are there.

The experience of sitting with the patient, keeping them company in the most profound sense, is a visible activity symbolizing the connections among all human beings. This is what the nurse experiences as well as the patient. It is this understanding that Carol H. referred to when she described waiting with the patient for death to arrive:

> I remember the first one who died who I was close to. . . . As I sat with him as he was dying, it reminded me of sitting with women in labor, giving birth. It's a very intimate experience. You don't know when it's going to happen, and you have to have the patience to wait for it. And it's momentous. It's happening and you have to give yourself to it.

Stephanie C. described it somewhat differently, but also emphasized the reciprocal nature of the relationship. She said:

> I've found that the patients come to you in a situation where everything is going on all at once, the past as well as the present and the future, the family, everything, history, the whole situation, and you bring all of that, too, of course, as a practitioner, and the meeting of these two in the middle, where you come together. I'm fascinated with this relational self, of both myself and the people that I'm dealing with. In the middle there, there's a kind of alchemy takes place. And it's like no other patient relationship, because every patient is unique. It's not always wonderful but it can be.

This is what these nurses look for in nursing and what they find in caring for patients with HIV disease. For them, the pleasure of nursing lies in this reciprocal exchange. The rituals of care relate the nurse to the patient as much as they relate the patient to the nurse. Bob G. agreed:

> It's almost like we're players on a stage, and here's a PCP pneumonia and a person, and I'm going to fulfill a role; I'm a nurse, and he's a person, and he's a person and I'm a person. We're going to work out

> this problem somehow, and we interchange and it's a holy thing. There's something that I can give and we can communicate between each other. It's just a wonderful thing that happens, and it's something that comes about in nursing practice, in that practice of nursing a patient, of enabling them to find what they have to do.

In these encounters, the nurse's perspective dovetails with the patient's perspective. Together they create a common ground. Despite their differences, they "co-exist across the same world" (Spiegelberg 1976: 556) and they become collaborators. Merleau-Ponty describes the experience of such interrelated subjectivities thus: "I am liberated from myself . . . I lend him [the other] my thoughts and he makes me think in turn" (quoted in Spiegelberg 1976: 556). The barriers come down, whatever the barriers might be that separate people, and a state of "pure focus, of inner unity and harmony" (Lifton 1979: 25) is achieved. It is in these moments that nurses and their patients transcend death as they experience timelessness together.

What these nurses work at creating in their practice is a space within which they and their patients can operate freely and simply as human beings. By ignoring the ephemeral criteria that distinguish one set of human beings from another, and by focusing on what connects every human being to another, they transcend a particular time and place. Their interactions acquire timelessness and they find themselves expressing eternal verities. In such experiences,

> the restrictions of the senses—including the sense of mortality—no longer exist. Poetically and religiously this has been described as "losing oneself." It can occur not only in religious or secular mysticism but also in song, dance, battle, sexual love, childbirth, athletic effort, mechanical flight, or in contemplating works of artistic or intellectual creation. This state is characterized by extraordinary psychic unity and perceptual intensity. (Lifton 1976: 43)

For nurses, experiences of transcendence occur when they perform those eternal gestures of human connection, those actions of physical care that contain within them the acknowledgment of a common humanity. These incidents of connectedness can be full of emotion. As Eliade said:

> Every time distrust, enmity, the struggle for life, . . . seems to me to be abolished—even if only for an instant—a powerful and obscure emotion takes over inside me, as if the actual condition of man and of the world were canceled and the paradisiac epoch glorified by

> the primitive myths [when the cosmos was one] were reestablished. (Quoted in Girardot and Ricketts 1982: 11)

In a practice that confirms the unity of mankind and the cosmos, the nurse acts in accordance with the moral precepts of the profession, and in so acting, feels in touch with the best part of the self. It makes nurses feel thoroughly alive. Rhonda P. described it this way:

> People talk about nurses being wonderful saintly people, but that isn't what it is. You get so much from what you do. I'll give you an example. Not too long ago, I decided that I hadn't done enough patient care recently, and I needed a fix. So we got a patient who was dying, and it was a complicated transfer. She came from another state, but they couldn't take her right away at the hospice here, so we were taking care of her for a while, and we couldn't find a nurse, so I said, "I'll go." Now, she was actively dying, and she was staying with her brother and her sister. She was in an enormous amount of pain, but the two days that I spent with her were, and please understand the way I use this word, wonderful. I did so much for her. I kept her comfortable. I talked to her sister and her brother about her death, about what that would be like. I prepared them for it. I did all the things that made me feel good. I was exhausted when I left there, but I was on such a high, [because of] what I had been able to do, and the difference that I made. I guess that's what it's all about. It's creativity. It's like nothing else. You're making something and you're making it better. There has never been anything else like it for me. Never.

What these comments express is the power and pleasure nurses experience as they practice nursing. Conceptualizing nursing as simply taking care of people is only half of the story. Nursing is also about nurses, about how they know what they need to know, and how what they know can be the foundation for a particular way of being in the world.

Chapter 11
Contemplative Cognition

To be a nurse like those in this study, a practitioner has to be able to know the patient well, because nursing looks at how disease is manifest in the individual. The course that the nurse will devise for the care of a patient depends on the individual's reactions. Therefore, nurses have to learn how to assess a patient clearly and intelligently.

The goal is not to identify with the patient. The goal is understanding. This understanding is achieved through a particular kind of openness to the "other," which in turn depends on a special form of cognition. This cognition utilizes sensory information, including both the patient's and the nurse's observations of bodily changes and processes, together with intellectual analysis and emotional responsiveness. Empirical observation, intellectual knowledge, and sensitivity to the psychological, emotional, cultural, and social factors affecting the patient's situation are all necessary if the nurse is to understand and respond appropriately to the patient's needs.

Patricia Benner (1984) describes this process as being "present" for the patient, but it is more than noting facts or performing operations. It means being aware of subtle changes, anticipating problems, keeping tabs on all that is happening and all that might happen. It means operating at a level of skill that is not explicit but which rests on extensive, concrete, practical experience. It includes the "gut feeling" highly skilled nurses have about what is happening to patients in their care. Marcia B. described it as "looking at people as a whole," something she said her nursing instructors trained her to do almost automatically:

> You have your instructor there saying, "Well, what's this going to do to this? What's the problem with the heart and the lungs going to do to the kidneys?" People are constantly making you [in nursing school] look at the whole picture, *which you can't see initially.* I often

> spent three or four hours before going into the ICU, often staying up until two in the morning, just trying to make sense of what was going on with patients. You have to try to make sense of it. Everything is involved. You have to be aware of how one thing reacts on another, and then reacts on social issues and family relations, and vice versa. (Emphasis added)

Nurses use their knowledge of science and medicine to determine the patient's physical condition, but they must also use other knowledge, including feelings and intuition, to ascertain the patient's emotional and psychological situation (Agan 1987; Sarter 1987). In this process, nurses must ignore their own prejudices and inclinations, without losing their own individuality.

Nursing process rests on this interaction, an interaction that depends on nurses' ability to be highly alert and responsive, both to the patient and to themselves. It is at the center of the meaning of "care." It is being attentive without being intrusive. It is being open without being passive. It is being cooperative without relinquishing autonomy.

This kind of nursing depends, in turn, on a particular kind of mental operation that is based on the capacity to "harmonize passion and idea" (Lifton 1979: 26). The nurse must be able to think *and* feel together with the patient. Benner (1984) speaks of being instrumental and expressive at the same time. Only then can the patient be known as an individual with the same dimensions and integrity as one knows oneself. This kind of knowledge is key to the practice of the nurses in this study and it rests on their ability to link thinking with feeling.

Such a mental operation can be thought of as the process of knowing concomitantly the subjective and objective status of the patient. It also takes note of the nurse's objective and subjective states. It thus combines two different viewpoints simultaneously. It is essential to the matching of perspectives that Merleau-Ponty describes in the encounter between two subjectivities (Spiegelberg 1976: 556). The practitioner is open to both viewpoints at the same time. As Benner says, "Nursing is a human science, conducted by self-interpreting subjects who are studying self-interpreting subjects, who *both* may change as a result of an investigation" (1984: 171; italics in original).

The kind of nursing practiced by the nurses in this study depends on their ability to comprehend and to incorporate the patient's perspective into a plan of care. This is achieved through a process I call contemplative cognition. In this process, myriad impressions register on the nurse's consciousness and have to be noted and sorted all at once. There is no particular sequence to the impressions received by the nurse, but many different kinds of information are absorbed and integrated. The physical condition of the patient, the patient's mental and emotional outlook, the patient's history, the patient's current situation—all of these aspects of the patient's status have to be understood in themselves and in relation to each other. At the same time, the nurse considers these factors against what she or he already knows about the patient and the illness. During this process, while directly focused on understanding the reactions and thoughts of the patient, the nurse is also aware of his or her own reactions and thoughts.

This process of understanding is similar to that often found in aesthetic, religious, and empathic experiences. These contexts are not totally analogous to the nursing situation and it would be unwise to treat them as such. Yet there are aspects of what happens in nursing that comparison with aesthetic and religious experience can illuminate. The sacred can be found in the mundane (Wolf 1988).

In aesthetic cognition, according to Watts and Williams, "one widely accepted tenet is that it involves a kind of distancing. We separate the object from ourselves" (1988: 60). The observer puts the object outside the sphere of his or her own personal concerns and of his or her own needs and desires, and by so doing, is able to look at it on its own terms. This is an essential part of nursing. The patient is the focus of the nurse's attention.

In order to do this, intellectual restraint is required. The observer cannot be distracted by extraneous thoughts or introspection. He or she cannot indulge in mental commentary on related matters. Associations with other objects must be suppressed, otherwise the primary object won't be seen clearly, and clarity is the first prerequisite for cognition. In addition, the observer must stop thinking of the past or the future and be centered in the present. The observer must also "reach out" to the object rather than remain absorbed in his or her own reaction to it. Contact must be sought. Thus knowledge combines with desire (Furth 1987).

This "reaching out" must include some feelings of affection or reverence, otherwise all that is achieved is a purely intellectual critical analysis of the object, not understanding. Jerome Bruner, in his essay on viewing the statue of the Virgin Mary in Toledo Cathedral, describes the torrent of emotional impulses he felt: he wanted to "father her, be mothered by her, make love to her, gossip with her, and just watch how the face will change when the child finally pokes her under the chin" (1962: 70). In just this way, the nurses in this study feel for their patients. Compassion pulls them toward their patients. They experience a "fellow feeling" for the sufferer (Gadow 1980), and thus emotion becomes a way to knowledge. As Benner says, there is "knowledge and wisdom to be gained from allowing emotions to direct attention and thoughts. Emotions are not viewed as 'interruptions'; they have significance and content in their own right" (1989: 97).

But here too restraint is called for. "Fellow feeling" in Gadow's phrase means that the nurse directs feeling toward the patient's joy or suffering, much as the observer of art focuses on the object. It does not mean that the nurse becomes one with the patient. Indeed, the nurse must be careful not to be carried away by his or her own feelings. If that happens, the experience becomes an exploration of the nurse, a self-analysis, not an appreciation of the patient. The nurse must work at being receptive without looking for any particular or immediate result. He or she has to let the event happen and must be careful not to become overly involved.

In religious cognition, the same mental and emotional faculties are used and in the same way. The religious person learns to focus his or her attention on God rather than on the self, and this attention is sustained and inspired by a love of God and a desire to know the deity. Attention is directed outside oneself, toward God.

Perhaps the best known exercise for religious knowing is the practice of meditation. In meditation the individual seeks to exclude the extraneous and to focus on what "exists in itself" (Watts and Williams 1988: 64). In Buddhist meditation, for example, as the novice works through a series of stages, his or her perception moves away from an analysis of actual physical phenomena toward a direct apprehension of form, contour, and texture. The result can be moments of illumination in which what is observed is discerned with directness and certainty. Such moments are difficult to describe except by reference to poetic language. In Jamesian terms, they are often ineffable and noetic, meaning full of knowledge but difficult to convey to others (James 1985 [1902]). E. Bullough has described these perceptions thus:

> When a work of art is successfully apprehended in appreciation the new aesthetic object which is actualised to awareness is perceived with more lucidity, as if a caul has been removed from in front of it. It is sharper and more vivid in detail as if it had been removed from the periphery to the focus of vision and it acquires a structure by which it is compacted into a unified configuration. (Quoted in Watts and Williams 1988: 61)

This is similar to the understanding nurses achieve of their patients. When all the information has been processed, the patient becomes clear. As the nurse comes to understand the perspective and history of the patient, the details coalesce into a pattern. Marcia B. described it this way:

> You don't get it right away. You have to experience it, you have to practice it. You might read about it to start, but eventually you don't have to think consciously, "What is this a part of?" You just know. You look at the patient, and you know. If it's an acute situation, you know what's going on, you almost don't have to think about it. It's not magic. It's your education and your ability to size up a situation real fast because you've seen it before. You don't have to think about the signs and symptoms of this problem. You just know it right away. You know what to do.

The ability to take the many discrete facts and perceptions about a patient and make sense of them depends on the same cognition that has been described for aesthetic and religious knowing. It is also an essential part of empathic knowing. Some commentators have even claimed that the practice of meditation develops the ability to empathize (Freedberg 1989; Watts and Williams 1988). Certainly, empathic knowing of other people has always been postulated upon vicarious emotional experience and the ability to see things from another person's point of view (Havens 1986). It also seems to be nonanalytical and intuitive. It is a way of being attuned to others while suspending judgment. It has sometimes been called "listening with the third ear" (Reik 1948).

Freud suggested that his students listen to their patients with an "evenly suspended attention" during which they were to avoid coming to conclusions or making judgments. The meaning of what the patients said would come clear in time and trying to force it into a preexisting frame of reference too early would cut off discovery (Watts and Williams 1988: 64).

The key to this kind of attention lies in being able to focus one's attention in such a way as to permit the free operation of the intelligence. One stops trying to force information into particular patterns and waits instead for a pattern to emerge spontaneously. As Simone Weil said:

> Attention consists of suspending our thought, leaving it detached, empty and ready to be penetrated by the object; it means holding in our minds, within reach of this thought, but on a lower level and not in contact with it, the diverse knowledge we have acquired. Our thought should be in relation to all particular and already formulated thoughts, as a man on a mountain who, as he looks forward, sees also below him, without actually looking at them, a great many forests and plains. Above all, our thought should be empty, waiting, not seeking anything, but ready to receive in its naked truth the object that is to penetrate it. (1973 [1951]: 111)

Weil describes this kind of attention in an essay on academic knowing, but she states that this kind of attention is also needed in order to know other human beings. It is certainly critical to the kind of nursing described in this study. It is an attention that allows practitioners to know their patients and to know themselves at the same time. But because they are not self-absorbed, they can direct their focus to the patient. They are concerned about the other's well-being. Thus their perception is open to feeling, because they direct their emotions as well as their intellect toward the patient.

This way of approaching others is central to how the nurses in this study practice. They try to set aside their own preconceptions and prejudices while making a sincere effort to absorb the point of view of the "other." Firm conclusions must not be reached too early. Rather, what has been learned is allowed to filter through their consciousness until the significance of what has been seen and heard becomes apparent.

A kind of "evenly suspended attention" is also essential to nursing. Nurses must be attentive but must resist being drawn too far into the patient's world. Yet at the same time they must be able to imagine what that world is like. The capacity to imagine another's position and experience, to imagine another's reaction to one's own actions, to imagine the next need and to anticipate it, this capacity facilitates nursing care. Bob G., who said he spent much of his time listening to patients, went on to say:

> It [nursing] is trying to throw away my preconceptions; it's sitting down and trying to define problems in a mutual way with the patient. It's asking them. I act as a reflector and what they say comes to me, and sometimes I try to order it so it helps them conceptualize in their mind what's going on. Sometimes I'll offer a suggestion or I'll try to offer choices. That's on an intellectual level. Sometimes it's just a hand on a shoulder. They need someone to touch them.

By combining clinical knowledge with emotional sympathy, the nurse is able to act in a way that will relieve the patient's discomfort, whether that discomfort is physical, social, or psychological. Jacques Maquet calls this thinking "contemplation." He says: "The contemplative mode of consciousness cannot be reduced to cognition; neither can it be reduced to affectivity" (1986: 166). It is nonlinear, creative thinking that meshes reason and emotion (Furth 1987).

Such thinking is central to the provision of care. To care for someone else is to process many kinds of information, including one's own feelings and thoughts. Out of a conglomeration of information, that "buzzing, blooming confusion" that William James (Girardot and Ricketts 1982) called life, the caregiver perceives a coherent pattern or picture of what is happening to a particular patient. When the picture is complete, when enough information has been gathered, the patient is seen with clarity. Then decisions about how to care can be made. Yet ideally the nurse's own ego is not involved. The other person has priority. As Havens says, "The full experience of noninvasive closeness awaits the development of a capacity to stand undistorted near those who shine forth fully on their own" (1986: 85).

In Maquet's words, "The beholder's ego is not the conquering ego of action, the assertive ego of [pure] cognition, the introspective ego of affectivity. It is the disappearing ego of contemplation" (1986: 165). Thus, in reaching out to the patient, the nurse can attain "a true and authentic transcendence of [the] self" (Gadow 1980: 91). Yet, as we have seen, such a transcendence brings with it intense feelings of being. Paradoxically, in contemplative cognition, the self is lost and regained.

In this kind of nursing, understanding is based on personal experience, the experience of meeting the unfamiliar and making it familiar. To do this the unfamiliar must first be construed as worth investigating. The outcome must be seen as valuable. The nurse must approach the investigation with a minimum of preconceptions and prejudices and abundant sympathy and interest. The nurse's individuality is subordinated to the patient's because the focus is on the "other." It is the patient's story that is important. The patient's views must be solicited and integrated with information from other sources. Finally, the assessment of the patient depends in some measure on the personal attributes, background, interests, and ambitions of the nurse. To be successful, a nurse needs, in Haven's felicitous phrase, to "combine modesty with authority" (1986: 103).

In nursing, knowledge of the "other" is the gateway to understanding. This is a kind of knowledge that is personal and infused with feeling. It is different from scientific knowledge. As Merleau-Ponty points out: "Science manipulates things and gives up living in them. It makes its own limited models of things; it operates upon these indices or variables to effect whatever transformations are permitted by their definitions. It comes face to face with the real world only at rare intervals" (1969: 252).

Science is concerned with making general laws that facilitate prediction and its object is "to reduce empiricism" (Bruner 1969: 74). That is exactly what the kind of nursing described in this study is not about. Nursing uses scientific knowledge—it needs science, it contributes to scientific knowledge—but it is not science in Merleau-Ponty's definition, a definition that removes science from the experience of physical life and from empirical experience.

Nursing, as practiced by the nurses I spoke with, does not try to escape from the empirical situation. On the contrary, it is within the empirical situation that the nurse finds the knowledge needed to care for the patient. Each nurse has her or his own knowledge of each patient. This knowledge is individual to the nurse. Yet it is knowledge that is used to construct a course of action, and it thus passes from the subjective to the objective. In this process there are always elements that remain ineffable, which cannot be communicated. Many particulars of how a conclusion was arrived at can be enumerated, but they do not, taken individually, add up to understanding. Still, understanding is there.

Michael Polanyi calls this kind of understanding "personal knowledge." With personal knowledge, we know that we know and we know what we know, but we cannot explain completely, or to another's satisfaction, how we arrived at our knowledge. As Polanyi says: "Although the expert diagnostician, taxonomist, and cotton-classer can indicate their clues and formulate their maxims, they know many more things than they can tell, knowing them only in practice, as instrumental particulars, and not explicitly, as objects" (1962: 88).

Not everyone has the talent or capacity for the kind of thinking that blends subjective and objective observation and which entails simultaneous awareness of oneself and others. It is a skill that must be learned, and it requires practice. Nurses usually learn this skill, if they learn it, in their practice. It is important to note, however, that nurses are not always engaged in intimate, intense, emotional and intellectual encounters with their patients. Contemplative cognition is not needed in every nursing encounter. But it is essential to nursing HIV-infected patients, and I believe that the nurses who are attracted to the care of HIV-infected patients do it well and enjoy doing it. It is what they are doing whenever they struggle to figure out the appropriate intervention for a particular patient. As Marcia B. said:

> You never know what's going to happen. You're trying to make a picture of the patient's symptoms. You ask yourself, "What is going on?" And you have to be good; you have to be able to pick up all the signs and symptoms and try to make a picture of them. Everyone's different and no one knows why some people develop one infection and others another; the reaction you see may be something more than a drug reaction. You have to keep everything in mind at once: who this person is, what their history is, your prior relationship, etc. etc. It's all important.

This is contemplative cognition. It is what these nurses are doing when they practice holistic nursing. The opportunity to engage in this kind of knowing is one of the attractions of this disease for these nurses, and the length of time HIV-infected patients spend under their care gives them opportunities to use and improve their skills.

Nurses who care for HIV-infected patients need to be adept at contemplative cognition for two reasons. The first is that HIV disease is a new disease and its natural progression is not yet definitively known. Indeed, it seems to manifest itself differently in different groups and in different countries (Harawi and O'Hara 1989). Nurses often have to rely on their own judgment with HIV disease, more so than with diseases more fully understood. Stephanie C. noted that "we're getting so good at keeping people alive that we're seeing weird infections that we never saw before, diseases doctors have only read about or haven't seen in that particular spot or this particular system, in different parts of the body."

The sense of being in unknown territory is strong. HIV-infected patients defy categories and expectations. As Gladys R. described it:

> With this disease especially, it takes so many turns. Right now we have lots of patients with MAI [mycobacterium avium-intracellulare]; it's a kind of TB, and these patients have very, very, very high fevers. They will be walking around saying "Hi" to us all, and I'll say, "What do you mean, 'Hi,' you've got a temperature." "Oh, I do?" they'll say. They don't even feel it, because their immune system is gone, and so they're not fighting it, so their body doesn't react to it. We had a woman whose temperature went up to 108 degrees. For men, I have never really seen too many men go beyond 106.

Because HIV disease is continually changing its manifestations, nurses have no script to rely on. As Marcia B. explained:

> You can't predict what's going to happen. You cannot predict your day. You always have to be flexible and change around, prioritize what you do for the day, you have to be flexible because anything can happen. And if you're rigid, you could never do it. Plus you also have to accept other people's lifestyles, and if you're rigid, you might not be able to do that. AIDS patients are challenging, they really are. They're depressed, they're afraid, they're emotionally needy. They need it all.

A nurse committed to HIV care must be good at observation, must enjoy the intellectual puzzle of coping with something unknown, must be self-aware yet self-effacing, and must feel for her patients. Such a nurse is close but distant, engaged but disengaged, sympathetic but restrained. These are contradictory demands, and satisfying them is the hardest thing nurses do. It means being true to oneself and to others at the same time.

Achieving this state of balance is difficult and difficult to sustain over time. Not infrequently, nurses find their ability to engage others in this way decreases as time goes on. Because this process must be repeated with each patient, nurses get tired and lose their energy. It may also be a capacity that naturally ebbs and flows, so that nurses may be more or less capable of it at different periods of their personal and professional lives.

This may be one reason that nurses change positions so frequently. One nurse told me she moved every eighteen months. Moving provides nurses with respite. Many move back and forth between positions that involve intense patient contact and those that are more impersonal. Such a pattern was clearly visible in many of the work histories of the nurses in my study. One nurse moved from an inpatient AIDS unit to an ambulatory clinic to a day program to an administrative position in a hospital. Then, at the time of our second interview, she was about to return to clinic work. Another nurse worked for five years with HIV-infected patients in home care, and then took a position in epidemiology. At the time of our second interview, she said she was ready to go back to direct care of HIV-infected patients.

Another difficulty with the kind of practice these nurses espouse is that it can only go as far as the other permits it. As a result, it is a limited knowledge. It can't be hurried; the other sets the pace because the work is collaborative. And because patients do not always understand their role in the process, nurses can become frustrated. In addition, because the organization and ethos of the American medical system gives little more than lip service to this part of nursing's enterprise, nurses burn out.

The nurses I interviewed said that their way of understanding and relating to patients is only taught obliquely in nurses' training. Young nurses watch other nurses and incorporate what they like from what they see. This is both good and bad. As Cassie N. said:

> I think it [HIV care] attracts people who can do this. I don't think they're trained. I don't think that nurses in any school are given bedside manner classes on how to relate to patients, how to be emotional. You're always told the same thing: treat them with respect, blah, blah blah. You develop it on your own in clinical [prac-

> tice]. Nobody tells ——— to dance for her patients or tells us to sing for them, to make friends with them. It's not something you have to do. It's just something you do.

If the relationship with patients that these nurses describe is not taught specifically, it is liable to engender misunderstanding. Young nurses can become disillusioned when they first start working because they do not experience the kind of personal relationship they expect with their patients, particularly in hospital work. Yet their picture of the desirable personal relationship may be an immature or incomplete one. It may focus too much on expending and accepting emotion, whereas the experienced nurse uses feeling to expand her or his knowledge about the patient. It is emotion in discipline to the intellect. It is sympathy, not sentimentality.

The nurses in this study are, with a few exceptions, mature women and men with years of nursing experience. Almost all of them are "experts" in Benner's (1984) phrase. They understand how to control their emotions and how to use their emotions to achieve the desired end. That end is knowledge, not emotion. Their goal is to understand the patient. This is why nurses can say that "love," in the popular sense, is not what they do, but it may be what Merleau-Ponty meant when he speaks of "adult love" as taking "the other person as he is, at his distance and in his autonomy" (1969: 95). It is what Weil is describing when she says:

> The capacity to give one's attention to a sufferer is a very rare and difficult thing. Warmth of heart, impulsiveness, pity are not enough. . . . The love of our neighbor in all its fullness simply means being able to say to him: "What are you going through?" It is a recognition that the sufferer exists, not only as a unit in a collection, or a specimen from the social category labeled "unfortunate," but as a man, exactly like us, who was one day stamped with a special mark of affliction. (1973 [1951]: 114)

The nurses I interviewed are nurses who find, in the care of HIV-infected patients, an opportunity to meet patients on this level. In order to do so, they need to use all their nursing skills. Those skills are intellectual, emotional, and physical. It is through using them together, rather than singly or sequentially, that nurses come to understand their patients and how to care for them. Instead of privileging rational activity, which is what modern consciousness does, this kind of nursing gives equal weight to the information gained from physical contact and from emotions. It meshes the ability to be objective and analytical with the exercise of empathy and intuition. Yet it also insists on "hands on," direct contact with the patient.

This kind of nursing thus offers to its practitioners a way of being in the world that keeps the body, the mind, and the heart together. It demands of practitioners "a participation of the entire self, . . . a unifying and directing of one's entire self in relation to another's need" (Gadow 1980: 90). It is achievable only by nurses "who act out of an explicit self-unity, allowing no dimension of themselves to be exempt from the professional relation" (Gadow 1980: 90). It is because nursing *is* a unified experience of body, mind, and heart—and because it demands from its practitioners a similar unity—that it is so powerful and so pleasurable.

Chapter 12
Personal and Professional Integration

The encompassing conception of nursing that the nurses in this study profess is difficult to honor in the workplace, but caring for HIV-infected patients does offer many of these nurses an opportunity to put their ideals into practice. As Bob G. said:

> When I was in nursing school, I was told wonderful things by my professors, wonderful things about what a nurse can do. There was a tremendous sense of scope in what a person in nursing could do. And then to get out into the reality was something else. I worked in ER for six years, and saw the inhumanity that was going on, and I had very little contact with people who thought the way I did. I often got discouraged, but I think in this work, in the last year, with the talents I've got, I've found that what I thought in nursing school was possible *is* possible. My practice is validating my beliefs about nursing and my belief in myself and my belief in the talents I have. It's that validation that is so rewarding. (Emphasis in original)

The "wonderful things nurses can do" are not limited to HIV disease, but there are a number of reasons why nurses who want to practice with this ample reach are attracted to HIV care. First, nurses find in the care of HIV-infected patients an opportunity to develop a holistic practice, because HIV infected patients need many different kinds of services and attention. Thus it satisfies the desire of these nurses to develop a particular kind of practice. In addition, because HIV care lacks status within the health-care system, it attracts less institutional attention than other diseases. As a result, nurses in HIV care are given more autonomy and independence to develop their own practices.

The autonomy nurses find in HIV care takes several forms. As Bob G. went on to say:

> I guess it's because we make our own job. The way it evolved in the hospital, we're not even under Nursing. They don't control us. They don't have us doing QAs [Quality Assurances]; we don't have to go to the meetings on all those things. My boss is the nurse who started the program, and then there's the doctors, and they don't know much about nursing. They just leave it to us, "Okay, nurse, do your thing." They know it's valuable and they appreciate it. Whatever we can come up with, it's good in their view.

This attitude gives nurses the chance to experiment and innovate. A nurse who was going to be in charge of an ambulatory clinic for HIV-infected patients commented:

> It's not like blood pressure clinics where everything is set. Even though the idea of how to run a clinic has been developing for years—and we still have a lot to learn about the mechanics of it, we don't have a number machine, for example—still on things like patient education, we're way out in front.

Patient education is essential if the transmission of HIV disease is to be contained and/or halted, and through patient education, nurses can have an impact far beyond the individual case. But influencing people and promoting behavior changes are much more complicated than following correct protocols and established routines, important as these are. Developing approaches and programs that work calls for ingenuity, inventiveness, and imagination. The nurse quoted above detailed the various steps she would take when she was in charge:

> Right now, the clinic doesn't offer condoms. But I will put out condoms when I'm in charge. I will try to find folders and handouts for people; I will try to anticipate problems, about diarrhea, about nausea. I will have a little present for patients every week. I'd do the kinds of things which aren't being done now, which reflect what I have to offer.

The concept of what the nurse has to offer can be broad in HIV care, and it is up to the nurse to determine how much is offered. It's not just the clinical skills, it's other capacities as well. And foremost among those capacities is the capacity to feel. Agnes S. said with some wonder:

> We had a patient who was very, very anxious, and I always had the feeling that I could never please him. It didn't matter what I tried to do. He was real anxious and he became very angry and disagreeable;

> he wasn't making any friends at that point. But his lover was there to smooth ruffled feathers, and I got close to him and how he was feeling, and he was there when he [the patient] died. I saw him crying and I just felt like I had to cry and I had never been that way before. I had always been real strong and tough, but this softens you up.

Nurses' training can promote callousness if it prohibits the expression of feeling. According to Watson, the prevailing attitudes in much nursing education ignore the role emotion plays in the relationship between nurse and patient:

> This [the nurse's relationship to patient] depends on authenticity and honesty, on genuineness and sincerity. [These are] almost entirely absent in our educational and socializing experiences in the nursing profession. [They are] instead substituted with artificial aims of professionalism and scientism. (1988: 69)

Toby B. commented:

> When I was in school I was always told to be "professional," which means showing no emotion, neither anger nor sadness. I might be upset, I might be tearful, but I had to remove myself from the situation; I could go to the bathroom and cry. God forbid that I should ever show a patient I was compassionate, or that I felt for them, that I cared for them, or that this was affecting me.

The nurses I interviewed thought it was neither desirable nor possible to be such an automaton. Toby counseled the young student nurses under her tutelage to acknowledge their feelings, both positive and negative, for the patient. She said to them:

> "If you have feelings and emotions, then show them. [On] this floor more than any, you have the opportunity to do that. If you are sad enough to cry, there's no reason why you shouldn't cry with the patient." I do it. I go in there and cry. Sometimes I'm angry. Some patients just get me downright angry. They'll be rude and I'll say to them, "I didn't deserve that. I'm trying to help and you're pushing me away. You're yelling at me and being obnoxious." I had one patient who was very manipulative and difficult, so I said to him, "Nobody wants to take care of you. I've got fifty-five nurses on my staff and nobody wants to take care of you. I can see one person maybe having a personality problem but not fifty-five." He got better behaved, but I had to be very straight with him.

Being able to be honest with their patients and with themselves is an attraction for many of these nurses. One administrator who had worked in a private hospital before joining the municipal system commented that in the private hospital "nobody seemed to die, whereas here, if a member of the staff or someone's relative dies, a notice about the funeral service is put up in the elevator or on the bulletin board. Death isn't hidden."

This attitude extends to dealing with HIV disease. One nurse observed that with AIDS patients the issue of death was always there. She said that she was very "up front about death [with her patients]. They have AIDS and they are going to die; not right away, but they are going to die."

It is this honesty about death that enables nurses to focus on life. The journey toward death has begun, but on the way many good things can happen. Stephanie C. found that humor was essential, for the patient and for herself. Laughing at life's absurdities was good for her and her patients. She said:

> There are times when you have a lot of fun. Some of the patients are incredibly good at maintaining a sense of humor. I remember one patient who had lost the sight in one eye and he was dying. He was losing his faculties and he was getting one infection after another. He looked up at me one day as I said, "How are you?" And he said, "Oh, this is all getting so boring. Every day it's the same thing. First, I get up with a fever and then I throw up and then I have diarrhea." And he went on and listed his day. And we started laughing and holding hands and just going over the whole thing, and he just thought it was funny. I'll never forget him.

In nursing HIV-infected patients, these nurses find the freedom to be fully and humanly involved in their work. They bring their repertoire as people to their work. Just as they take a holistic view of the care their patients need, so they want to be able to bring all their faculties and talents to bear on the task of caring for HIV-infected patients. They become holistically involved themselves in their patients' care. They are not simply the technicians and clinicians. They are involved in their work as whole people, which Gadow suggests is a "necessary corollary for the optimal healing of their patients" (1980: xxv).

These nurses remember funny stories to tell their patients. They talk about movies they've seen or trips they've taken. They keep track of birthdays. They bring food and flowers to their patients. They sometimes get involved far beyond what other nurses might feel are the appropriate boundaries of care.

Gretchen S., for example, spent a great deal of time helping one of her patients arrange for custody of her children. Because her patient wanted to separate her children, giving one to her mother, one to her sister, one to an aunt, she consulted a friend who was a lawyer. The lawyer's opinion was that the judge would not approve this arrangement because it separated the children. Gretchen then went back to her patient and helped her devise another plan. Later, after the patient died, Gretchen found herself involved in complex negotiations with a funeral home and the New York City welfare department. The funeral home wouldn't pick up the body from the hospital until it received some money; the patient's family had no money; welfare had to go through channels before releasing the money. Meanwhile, the patient's body lay unclaimed.

The objective needs of many of HIV-infected patients match the subjective desire of these nurses to go beyond clinical requirements. Because so many HIV-infected patients lack family support, hospitals take on responsibilities once reserved for patients' families, and thus nursing HIV-infected patients can mean being involved in issues that used to be handled by family members. HIV disease has revealed how isolated and alone many people in American society are. Part of the goal of the nurses in this study is to demonstrate to HIV-infected patients that they are not alone.

In order to do this, the nurses in this study often go outside the strict limits of their "professional" role. Nurses who are willing to go this far for their patients frequently favor an open kind of practice. They respond on many different levels to their patients, and they recognize that their patients have a number of different responses to their disease. So, for example, they are frequently open to what non-traditional treatments may offer their patients. As Cassie N. said:

> You certainly learn a lot up here. You learn about alternative medicine. I have patients who believe in crystals. I have patients who believe in special machines and Chinese herbs. The way I feel about it is, as long as you don't give up on conventional medicine, whatever you want to add to it that's not harmful, that's fine. If you want to sleep with crystals on your chest, if you want someone to come in and spray incense in your room, that's all fine with me as long as you don't give up on conventional medicine. I've had people on macrobiotic diets, all of which are accepted by a great part of the community here. I've never found any of these things to work, but if they

> make you feel better and if they put your mindset in the direction of getting well, it's not going to hurt.

The nurses I interviewed were open to other perspectives because they could not cure, but sought to heal their patients. Patients would never be HIV free, but they could be restored to psychological wholeness, to a renewed sense of self, to revitalized living even though ill.

Whatever promotes this process is therefore good, whether it is strictly medical or not. It might mean incorporating mental imaging into a program or experimenting with electrical stimulation to alleviate peripheral pain. Part of the freedom HIV care offers to these nurses is the freedom to bring other therapies into the medical system. Because administrators and doctors give HIV units more latitude than other units, sometimes for compassionate reasons, nurses can experiment. They can respond with more than the traditional array of medications. And they can, if they like, respond with more of themselves than they could in another specialty in which protocols and therapies were more defined.

Responding personally means, in part, that the nurse is not afraid to reveal personal information to the patient. Some of the lines which are usually drawn between patient and caregiver are thereby erased. Bette V. used her artistic ability to create fantasy objects for her patients: "I like to do things with my hands. I draw and paint. It's a gift and a comfort, I think, for the patient." As Watson explains:

> The more of ourselves we do not have to exclude [from encounters with others], the more of the other we can be open to. Our self-awareness . . . and self-acceptance, our actualization of our potential, allows us to share with others so that they can *become* in relation to us. (1988: 5; italics in original)

This is holistic work, in which individuality becomes a therapeutic tool. In such work, the practitioner calls on a personal repertoire of knowledge as well as professional training. Stephanie C. said of what she was doing: "It has become very clear to me that I'm in the right place. I really feel that everything I've learned in my life, my whole inventory, and then some, are being put to use."

Such nursing requires courage, the courage to be open and to risk exposure. It means being ready to risk humiliation. The nurse may jeopardize the nursing enterprise by saying the wrong thing, making the wrong gesture, antagonizing or offending the patient. It can be a daunting prospect, and even those who feel a strong desire to work with HIV-infected patients, because it will let them practice this way, feel some trepidation as they begin. Maria J. said:

> I always felt that these [HIV-infected] patients' needs weren't being met. The fear of providers was enormous. Patients would die and no one would know what to do with the family. That's how I got into this. But when I got this job I wondered emotionally if I was going to be able to do it. If I couldn't do it emotionally, what good was I going to be to the patient? I thought about it for a week and I said, "I don't know if I can, but I want to do this so badly. I care so much. I'll give it a try and see how patients respond."

In this statement, we can see the ambivalence most nurses caring for HIV-infected patients experience at one time or another. The challenges seem too great, the rewards too meager. It is tempting to consider giving up. Nurses frequently move back and forth between exhilaration and discouragement. Some days are terrific, when progress seems assured. Some days are terrible, when progress stalls or decline begins. HIV disease is not only a rollercoaster for the patient; it is for the nurse also.

Yet the nurses I spoke with do stay with it, despite the difficulties. One reason they do is that HIV care offers them the chance to be themselves in their work. The work may be difficult, but the nurse wants to be there. As Maria J. went on to say:

> It's depressing, it is. The patients come and go and eventually they die. That's the hard part. But I feel a lot happier, a lot more satisfied now than I did when I was a general surgery nurse. I get to do a lot of teaching and spend a lot of time with the patients. You have to be so sensitive. You are required to spend more time with the patient. They feel better. I feel good about that.

Toby B. was even more emphatic: "This is the happiest and the most fulfilled I've ever felt in nursing, including the ICU, the ER, and anything else." It is satisfying because what the nurse has to offer and wants to offer is exactly what is needed. Paula T. added: "I'm where I'm needed, and I'm getting tremendous personal satisfaction from the knowledge that I'm competent and that I'm caring and that I have something to offer."

Nurses have always been competent and caring, but they have often been relegated to the background of the medical system. What a medical crisis on the order of HIV does is make visible how important nurses are. This was true during the Civil War, during the epidemics of the twentieth century, and during the military conflicts of recent memory.

What is also true today as was true in previous medical crises is that the health care system has not been able to cope with the challenge of the disease. There are not enough physical facilities, there is not enough medical knowledge, there are not enough people to do what has to be done. The procedures and protocols are not established. As a result, medical institutions have to relax their control, and, therefore, some of the antagonism between nursing and the institutional framework within which it operates subsides.

Nursing, like other predominantly female professions, draws its values from the private sphere of home and familial attachments, but the institutions within which nurses work are organized on public, bureaucratic, and universalistic principles. Nursing looks at the individual, focuses on need, and adjusts to circumstance. It is somewhat ad hoc. Hospitals and clinics and agencies are not.

They are, like all bureaucratic organizations, concerned with order and predictability. Standards are established that are to be applied across the board, and these standards are to be applied impersonally and with "affective neutrality" (Berger, Berger, and Kellner 1974: 52). Both caregiver and patient are assumed to be somewhat featureless and anonymous. The focus is on following the proper procedures, the means that will result in the desired end. The consciousness within the bureaucratic organization is one of abstract depersonalization. Emotion is controlled and directed.

> Bureaucracy assigns emotional states. The bracketing of personal bias, the objective assignment of cases into their appropriate boxes, the painstaking adherence to proper procedure even in situations of great stress—all of these are not just elements of cognitive style but presuppose specific emotional controls. (Berger, Berger, and Kellner 1974: 58)

For nurses whose values are different from those dominant in large organizations, the experience of working in bureaucratic organizations can be painful. So much of what they believe and what they seek to do is directly contrary to the fundamental principles underlying the institutions they work in. As Berger, Berger, and Kellner note:

> At least potentially, this constitutes a threat to the individual's self-esteem and, in the extreme case, to his subjective identity. . . . One may safely generalize here that the threat will be felt in direct pro-

> portion to the development of individualistic and personalistic values in the consciousness of the individual. Where such values are highly developed, it is likely that the intrinsic abstraction of bureaucracy will be felt as an acute irritation at best or an intolerable oppression at worst. . . . The individual whose allegiance is given to such values is almost certainly going to resent being treated "as a number." (1974: 56)

There is thus a fundamental contradiction between nursing and the institutions that hire nurses. It is this contradiction which working with HIV-infected patients reconciles. In HIV care, the institutional values take second place. Particularly in dedicated units, clinics, and agencies specializing in HIV-infected patients, institutional power is relaxed. Nurses can sometimes determine how their units run. Staffing and hours can be adjusted to the needs of the patients and the nurses. Nurses find that they acquire autonomy. As Cassie N. said:

> We're understaffed, but a lot of us do overtime, so that we can keep the unit staffed with people we know, and of course there are monetary benefits for those of us who do it all the time. There's no question about that, but when we first opened, we were relying on the hospital to give us nurses from a per diem pool, and they just couldn't meet our needs. So now we're trying to book our own, that is, we sign up for overtime knowing that we'll be on this unit, and it seems to be working better.

In many dedicated units, in clinics, and in home-care agencies devoted to HIV-infected patients, nurses can follow their own bent and institute a kind of nursing that is congruent with their principles and ideals. Thus some of the strain nurses commonly feel in their jobs is removed. Nurses can concentrate on what they like to do and what they're good at doing.

At the same time, in doing what they like to do, nurses in HIV care now find that their perspective is espoused by some members of the medical and political establishments. Until very recently, medicine treated all patients alike, with similar drugs and similar dosages for men and women, for blacks, Hispanics, whites, and Asians. Now there is a growing recognition that, because women have not been included in much medical research, the conclusions cannot be automatically extended to them. There is a further recognition that different ethnic groups have different vulnerabilities and respond differently to drugs. Medicine is becoming somewhat more nuanced, more subtle in its applications.

In this respect, it is moving closer to nursing, which has always said that the patient, as an individual, must be considered as well as the disease. In caring for HIV-infected patients, this convergence is not only more apparent but more necessary, since the disease expresses itself slightly differently in each patient. Thus, for the nurses involved in HIV care, another source of tension and conflict is diminished. Nursing's viewpoint is validated. Individual doctors are still difficult, policies are still restrictive, but in some important ways, in HIV care, medicine itself is less monolithic than it once was and more receptive to nursing. As Chris T. commented: "One of the things I think AIDS has done within the medical system is loosen the boundaries between the professions and between the role descriptions. It provides an opportunity for people to grow professionally."

Particularly in AIDS units, where the physicians and the nurses have made a commitment to work with HIV-infected patients, there can be a close working relationship. As Alice D. said:

> If you have a good working team, a team which works well together, if you have a doctor and a nurse and you include a social worker and a psychologist and whatever, perhaps the clergy, and whoever else is appropriate, and you work together, you try to come up with some kind of game plan that is best for the patient, consulting them, too, including them in on what they want. In a good team, there's a great deal of respect for each other.

In addition, this kind of nursing's emphasis on the patient and its focus on the idiosyncratic expression of disease aligns it squarely with the dominant values of American society. Concepts of individual choice and notions of self-direction are central to HIV care. The nurses I interviewed were unanimous in placing the right for final decisions about treatment with the patient. This is consonant with the stress American society places on autonomy and independence. Patients are to be given the right to choose. They are to agree to treatment. Decisions are not to be made for them. This is an anti-authoritarian and egalitarian viewpoint.

The nursing practiced by the nurses in this study also finds an echo in the three major political movements of the past thirty years, the civil rights drive and the gay liberation and women's movements, all of which emphasized individual rights. Supporting the patient's right to be the final arbiter is consistent with the political philosophy of these causes. In New York City, with its liberal political traditions, these are powerful forces. For nurses caring for HIV-infected patients, this means that they can work without feeling that they are all on their own.

In Peter Berger's terms, they are not in the position of a "cognitive minority, a group of people whose view of the world differs significantly from the one generally taken for granted in their society" (1974: 6). They may have to defend their point of view, but they have the comfort of knowing that, no matter what the individuals they have to struggle with believe, there are many other people in the New York area who see issues as they do.

A crisis frequently calls into question ordinary ways of doing things. What has been taken for granted is often examined anew. In the nursing of HIV-infected patients, this examination has reaffirmed the validity and value of nursing's traditions, most particularly its concentration on the individual. Nursing has always functioned on this basis, but only recently has the congruence between nursing's values and overarching communal values become so apparent. Nursing's point of view is compatible with general American values of autonomy and independence. And, in New York City, nurses committed to the care of HIV-infected patients have the support of prevalent political and social attitudes.

Thus, in responding to HIV disease, the nurses I interviewed are being true to themselves, to their profession, and to their social beliefs. Because the institutions they work in have relaxed some of their control, these nurses can respond to the disease according to their own scale of values. As a result, HIV nursing is a specialty in which there is less tension than in most occupations between what produces success professionally and success personally. Strategies that support honesty, sincerity, and authenticity, which are personal virtues, are not at variance with the strategies necessary for professional competence. For these nurses, in this work, the personal, professional, and political are in harmony, not in conflict. It is this congruence, that makes HIV care so attractive and so satisfying to the nurses I interviewed. For these nurses, the care of HIV-infected patients is indeed a special world.

Chapter 13
Images of Care

The images of themselves that the nurses in this study hold are images of physical care and connection. Patients are in bed, nurses are sitting by them, holding their hands, listening as they speak, responding in turn. Sometimes nurses and patients move side by side, linked arm in arm. In every setting, nurse and patient touch. This is emblematic of the contact that must also occur in other domains as well if the nurse and patient are to work together.

Even for nurses who are male, the image of the nurse can be an image of a woman. Certainly the behavior represented in the image is that associated with women, since it is the mother in American society who is responsible for the physical care of children and family members who are ill. Perhaps that is why the male nurse quoted earlier said of his own image of a nurse: "It's funny, really, I'm a man, but I picture nursing as someone in a white uniform, a woman bending over a bed, soft lights, the whole works."

Images of nurses held by the general public in American culture are usually of female figures. Indeed, the preponderance of women in the profession and its genesis within household responsibilities have tempted some to suggest that femaleness and nursing are archetypically linked. Woman equals Nurse and Nurse equals Woman are familiar equivalences in the popular mind (Fiedler 1988). This easily moves on to another equivalence: Woman equals Mother, and thus Nurse equals Mother.

It may be, however, that the image of the nurse as a female has less to do with biology and more to do with the fact that it is within relationships with women that members of American culture experience the personal attention that is at the center of care. It is also generally within the domain of domestic life in America, a domain under female control, that this kind of relationship is learned and practiced. Therefore, a female figure is used to represent this kind of a relationship because it brings with it the ideas of care and attention. Nurses are not mothers, but they sometimes act like mothers, and their patients sometimes act like children. It is this analogy that the image seeks to project, bringing diverse domains together through the representation of a female. There are male nurses, too, but the male figure in American culture does not elicit the same response. Therefore a male figure bending over the patient does not come automatically to mind when nursing is pictured.

Personal care in American culture *is* the province of women, and so images of nurses as women reflect social reality. Women are the caregivers in American society, and they are socialized more than men are in the skills of empathic understanding. They are taught more directly, more concretely, and more completely than men, to "think of others." As a group, therefore, they are more apt to come to nursing with some of the skills needed in a profession based on personal relationships. Whether socialization builds on a natural propensity is open to question, since the answer to such a question depends on a group of men being raised as women. It is true, however, that women are more likely than men to be able to use imagination and emotion as a pathway to knowledge, because their social role in American society has been largely defined in affective terms (Belenky et al. 1986; Jagger 1989; Keller 1985; Tronto 1990).

When nurses' training emphasizes a holistic approach to the patient, nurses are encouraged to consider and use emotion as a mechanism for understanding the patient. They expect to incorporate feeling into practice and so may seek in their work the kind of convergence of emotion and thought which the nurses I interviewed speak of finding in the care of HIV-infected patients. These expectations, expectations about the integration of thought and feeling, are very much at variance with the organization of work in American society. It requires distinct divisions between public and private repertoires of expression and thought. Nurses' training encourages integration; work in a technological and industrial society discourages it and, instead, promotes fragmentation.

In HIV care nurses can escape fragmentation. They find an opportunity to bring together in their work their intellectual, moral, affective, and social worlds. In this kind of nursing, all these domains become one. The meshing of domains, for the patient and the nurse, is what holistic nursing is all about.

Being involved in HIV care is also a way of being fully a part of the historical moment. HIV infection is a particular disease at a particular moment of time. The nurses in this study each have a particular history that they bring to their work. Nursing has a history, too. The treatment of illness, and the treatment of the poor, minorities, homosexuals, and so forth—these all have histories in America. These elements come together in the care of HIV-infected patients, so that the playing out of the drama of HIV disease is, in part, a playing out of social as well as individual narratives.

It is this complexity that provides the richness of caring for HIV-infected patients. For the nurses in this study, their work is an opportunity to live fully and to live out some of the major social issues of our time. They see what they are doing reflected in the media, in professional journals, and in political debates. They are part of one of the central dramas of our century.

In addition, they find that all their knowledge and all their skills, personal and professional, are needed to care for HIV-infected patients. This is not what most workers find in their jobs. It is certainly not something that the institutions that hire nurses are concerned about. Nor is it something that the health-care system as a whole strives to make possible for any caregiver.

What has made possible the integration of personal and professional here is the coming together of a number of elements: First is the nature of HIV disease and the particular populations it brings to the medical system; second is the relaxation of institutional oversight by hospital and medical personnel, along with the establishment of specialized, relatively autonomous HIV programs, and third is the desire on the part of these nurses to practice holistically.

This last point may be the most important. For these nurses, the practice of their profession has become an expression of their humanity. It may also be the discovery of what being a human being means. Certainly it lets them experience psychological wholeness, because to care for HIV-infected patients is to draw on all one's reserves of intelligence, emotional empathy, and physical strength. Cognitive, affective, and physical skills are required all at the same time.

What HIV disease has done for this particular group of nurses is provide them with a context for vitalization, both personally and professionally. The challenge of HIV disease to a society lulled into complacence lies in making clear the ambiguities and uncertainties of human life. In responding to this challenge, these nurses have found security in insecurity and certainty in uncertainty by relinquishing demands for ultimate answers. Instead, they turn to other human beings and find in their commitment to them an answer to the unknowns in human life, what Fernandez (1982) calls the "dark at the bottom of the stairs."

The images these nurses have of nursing embody this answer. To the terror that HIV disease provokes, these nurses reply with images of connection, of people helping other people, of direct person-to-person contact. These images express what to the individual may be inchoate and unformed. Within the image of the figure by the bedside, the listening posture, the helping hand, the ideal relationship and the ideal behavior are delineated. These are collective representations symbolizing mankind's ties to others and to human history, past and to come.

By embracing and validating these images, by using them as guides to action, these nurses defeat death by focusing on that which lives on forever, as long as the human species survives and as long as humanity remembers what being human requires (Lifton 1976). Within these images lies the meaning of the nursing profession. The profession itself is sustained through them.

The meaning of these images is that life is a unitary experience of body, mind, and emotion. Because human life is bodily, it is not eternal, nor can it be free of pain. Yet, paradoxically, by accepting that human life must end, a way is found to express what can transcend pain and sorrow, the recognition of another's humanity. And, because this understanding of human life is rooted in an acceptance of the body, it is fitting that it should be expressed in images of bodily human contact.

For the nurses I interviewed, the images they hold of nursing express the assumptions and values of their profession and so provide a basis for concerted action. By holding these images in common, these nurses have a standard against which to judge their own and others' performances. These images constitute a cultural frame within which is created an "imagined community" (Anderson 1983), a community which relies on these images for support and sustenance.

It is a community of all those who accept these images. It is a community with elastic boundaries, a community of people who do not have to live near each other or speak the same language to feel connected. Of the nurses I interviewed, only a few know each other as more than colleagues. The others are acquaintances or strangers. They have diverse backgrounds, diverse educations, diverse experiences. But they come together as nurses, nurses committed to a particular kind of nursing, made visible in the images they hold of human connection. To the extent that they give allegiance to these images, these nurses have created a confraternity that transcends differences, differences among themselves and between them and their patients.

In creating a framework within which their patients can be accepted as they are, these nurses apply the same standards to themselves. The openness and accessibility that they offer to their patients they also offer to themselves. For their patients and for themselves, the nursing encounter becomes an exercise in freedom, an opportunity to ignore all those distinctions that erect barriers between people, and to focus instead on what draws them together. In honoring their patient's humanity, they honor their own.

They see themselves reflected back from their patients. Their patients act as mirrors, but the reflection is not exact, and their perception is selective. Nurses can choose to see some things and not others. The nurses in this study choose not to see the poverty, the disarray, the despair, the failure. They choose to see courage and strength. They define the image of themselves that they see in their patients.

The appeal of caring for HIV-infected patients lies in this mutuality. The nurses in this study practice as they do because they believe in a particular philosophy of care. Their philosophy of care is founded on a moral stance according to which every human being is worthy, and thus worthy of care. In striving to maintain this code, the nurses I interviewed learn who they are and who they might become. They experience moments of transcendence when they succeed in making their code a reality. They are transformed through their contact with the transformations of their patients. Thus they experience that wholeness of mind and body that is the essence of healing, illustrating the dictum that what we do for others, we do also for ourselves.

Appendix A: Interview Guide

In drawing up this interview guide, my intention was to frame questions as broadly as possible so that the nurse could respond from the context of her or his own experience. I always began the interview with the first two questions; the others I covered as the conversation developed. But in each interview every topic was broached and discussed.

1. What do you do?
2. How did you come to nurse HIV-infected patients?
3. Do you remember your first HIV-infected patient?
4. Do you find HIV-infected patients different from other patients?
5. Do they require more of you?
6. What are the challenges of what you do?
7. What are the satisfactions?
8. Do you think there are ethical issues in what you do?
9. Do you get to know your patients well? Is this something you look for in your job?
10. Do you discuss your concerns with others (family, friends, colleagues, administrators, etc.)? What do they say?
11. Do you have any particular image of nursing? Any particular thing which, when you think of yourself as a nurse, you picture yourself doing?
12. What do you think nursing should be?
13. Would you recommend nursing to young people today?
14. Do you think there are aspects of HIV disease, or of the public's response to it, which make taking care of HIV-infected patients more difficult than caring for other patients?
15. If you were organizing AIDS care, would there be anything you would do differently?
16. Do you think your colleagues in the health-care system understand the nurse's job?

17. What do you think nurses' expectations of nursing are, and do they conflict in the care of HIV-infected patients?
18. What is your view of the issue of "Who is in control"?
19. What sustains you as you do this work?
20. Do you expect to continue to care for HIV-infected patients?

Appendix B: Survey of Nurses in AIDS Care

Responses

The numbers given represent those who indicated that the listed response was important. The percentage of the total is given in parentheses. The total was greater than fifty-six (the number of respondents) when more than one answer was given.

1. *What prompted you to become involved in HIV care?*

   Desire to help: 39 (69%)
   Desire to use skills/talents: 33 (58%)
   Intrigued with disease: 29 (51%)
   Personal contact with disease: 13 (23%)
   Attractive job: 11 (19%)
   Other—AIDS unit opened: 6 (10%); commitment to community: 3 (5%); wanted change: 3 (5%)

2. *What are the challenges of what you do?*

   Patients' emotional needs: 48 (85%)
   Comforting patients and families: 39 (60%)
   Coping with patient deterioration—physical: 32 (57%); mental: 33 (58%)
   Patients' clinical instability: 32 (57%)
   Working with colleagues who do not share your philosophy of care: 32 (57%)
   Coping with death: 32 (57%)
   Sustaining patients' hope: 31 (55%)
   Overcoming bureaucratic obstacles: 31 (55%)

Social stigma of disease: 26 (46%)
Maintaining own emotional balance: 24 (42%)
Working within limitations of care: 20 (35%)
Persevering through difficulties and failure: 16 (28%)
Coping with contagion: 8 (14%)
Other—keeping up with current knowledge: 2 (3%); placing terminally ill patients and children of HIV patients in hospices and homes: 2 (3%); reaching noncompliant patients: 2 (3%); disdain from colleagues and friends: 2 (3%).

3. *What are the satisfactions?*

Teaching and counseling: 43 (76%)
Involvement in important work: 42 (75%)
Establishing a personal connection with patients: 41 (73%)
Being able to use every kind of nursing skill: 36 (64%)
Meeting the challenge of clinical care: 32 (57%)
Working with like-minded colleagues: 27 (48%)
Other—helping patients face death and unfinished business: 3 (5%); facing the possibility of death for myself: 2 (3%); opportunity to be gentle and compassionate: 1 (2%).

4. *Do you meet any ethical issues in your work?*

Access to treatment/drugs: 35 (63%)
DNRs (Do Not Resuscitate orders): 30 (53%)
Termination of treatment: 29 (51%)
Recognizing the limits of high-tech medical care: 29 (51%)
Maintaining confidentiality: 28 (50%)
Toxic medication: 25 (44%)
Notifying partners/family members: 20 (35%)
Encountering suicide requests: 19 (32%)
Pregnancy decisions by HIV+ patients: 15 (26%)
Other—physicians and institutions uninterested in care of patients: 3 (5%); cost of care and medication: 1 (2%); conflicts between patients' wishes and their families': 1 (2%); fear of HIV patients in at-risk population: 1 (2%).

5. *What keeps you going?*

Pleasure from patient contact: 45 (80%)
Feeling that work is meaningful/needed: 44 (78%)

Personal growth: 36 (64%)
"Making a difference": 36 (64%)
Commitment to providing health care for all: 36 (64%)
Helping others: 30 (53%)
Clinical interest: 30 (53%)
Having interests outside work: 23 (40%)
Feeling of identification: 11 (19%)
Support from family and friends: 11 (19%)
Other—belief in God: 1 (2%); working with like-minded colleagues: 1 (2%); appreciation from patients: 1 (2%).

6. Do you have a support group at work?

Yes: 29 (51%)
No: 27 (48%)
If no, would you like one?
Yes: 11 (19%); No: 9 (16%)
No response: 7 (12%).

7. How long do you expect to be in HIV care?

1–3 years: 4 (7%)
3–5 years: 5 (8%)
5+ years: 2 (3%)
Indefinitely: 30 (53%)
Not sure: 12 (20%)

8. Are you concerned about becoming infected through patient contact?

HIV: 14 (25%)
TB: 27 (48%)
Pneumonia: 3 (5%)
Other—hepatitis: 4 (6%); Salmonella: 1 (2%).

9. How do you think about death?

A final end: 9 (16%)
A passing to another kind of existence: 39 (69%)
Other—peace and fulfillment: 4 (7%); union with God: 2 (3%)
No response: 2 (3%).

10. When you think of being a nurse, does a particular image come to mind, such as:

Listening as a patient talks: 42 (74%)
Talking with a patient: 39 (69%)
Giving physical care: 31 (55%)
Sitting by a patient's bed, holding his/her hand: 27 (48%)
Walking arm and arm with the patient: 20 (35%)
Dispensing medications: 20 (35%)
Other—being there for patients: 11 (19%); conferring with doctors, other health-care providers: 3 (6%).

11. Has HIV affected your relations with doctors?

Improved collaboration and collegiality: 38 (67%)
Increased your autonomy: 39 (69%)
Brought you into conflict: 24 (42%)
If so, on what issues?—treatment goals: 13 (23%); death/DNRs: 5 (9%); incompetence: 3 (5%); homophobia: 3 (5%); confidentiality: 1 (2%); issues of care for women and children: 1 (2%)
How do you handle them?—information gathering: 12 (21%); assertiveness/confrontation: 6 (10%); discussion and advocacy: 9 (16%).

12. Has HIV affected your relations with officialdom/bureaucrats/administrators?

No difference: 16 (28%)
Positively: 6 (10%)
Negatively: 22 (39%)
No response: 12 (21%)
If so, please describe:
Positive effect—openness and respect: 5 (9%); forced accountability and ethical decision-making: 1 (2%)
Negative effect—pressure to shortchange patients in the name of efficiency: 13 (23%); insensitivity to patient's needs: 9 (16%); difficulty getting through red tape: 4 (8%); disagreements over staffing levels: 11 (19%); discrimination against HIV patients: 3 (5%); "playing games with people's lives": 1 (2%).

13. What prompted you to become a nurse?

Desire to take care of the sick: 29 (51%)
Always wanted to be a nurse: 23 (40%)

Ideal of service: 17 (30%)
The many different careers in nursing: 16 (28%)
Interest in medicine: 15 (26%)
Job security: 12 (21%)
One of few career choices available: 10 (17%)
Nurses in family: 7 (12%)
Other—parental pressure: 3 (5%); interest in women's health: 1 (2%); a "people" profession: 1 (2%); army experience: 1 (3%); no particular reason: 4 (8%).

14. *Were you influenced in choosing nursing by books about nurses, such as biographies of Florence Nightingale?*: 8 (14%)

Clara Barton: 8 (14%)
Movies: 2 (3%)
TV shows: 3 (5%)
Others—biographies of Lillian Wald: 2 (3%); Rose Hawthorne: 1 (2%); Mary Anne Bickerdyke: 1 (2%) Cherry Ames novels: 5 (9%).

15. *Would you recommend nursing to young people today?*

No: 13 (23%)
Yes: 46 (82%)
Why "no"?—long hours and hard work: 6 (10%); low status, low salary: 4 (7%); high stress: 2 (3%); little power: 2 (3%); not creative: 1 (2%); little appreciation: 1 (2%)
Why "Yes"?—personal growth and satisfaction: 11 (19%); variety: 9 (16%); intellectual excitement: 5 (8%); chance to be creative and caring: 5 (8%); opportunities to make changes: 4 (7%); economic security: 4 (7%); worthwhile "real world" profession: 3 (6%); improving salaries 3 (6%).

TABLE B.1. Demographic information of respondents.

	No. of respondents	*Percent*
Age (years)		
20–30	0	0
30–40	30	53
40–50	19	32
50+	7	12
Years of nursing experience		
1–3	0	0
3–5	3	2
5–10	8	14
10–15	20	35
15–25	15	26
25+	9	16
No response	1	2
Degree(s)		
Diploma	8	14
Associate	5	8
B.A.	19	32
B.S.	24	42
M.S./M.A.	22	39
M.S./M.A. in progress	4	7
Ph.D.	2	3
No response	4	7
Current job		
Staff nurse	10	17
Clinician	20	35
Coordinator/director	8	14
Educator	6	10
No response	12	21
Years in current job		
0–1	9	16
1–3	17	30
3–5	10	17
5–10	6	10
10+	2	3
No response	12	21

TABLE B.2. Demographics of respondents' patient population.

	Percent of respondents' patient population	*Number of respondents*	*Percent of respondents*
Male patient	100	1	2
	90–99	15	26
	80–89	4	7
	70–79	6	10
	60–69	7	12
	50–59	7	12
	40–49	2	3
	0	5	8
Female patient	100	2	3
	90–99	1	2
	60–69	1	2
	50–59	4	7
	40–49	6	10
	30–39	5	8
	20–29	7	12
	10–19	14	25
	1–9	7	12
	0	4	7
Child patient	100	1	2
	90–99	1	2
	80–89	1	2
	20–29	1	2
	10–19	6	10
	1–9	3	5
	0	38	67
	(no response)	5	8
Race/ethnicity			
White	90–99	6	10
	80–89	1	2
	70–79	2	3
	60–69	5	8
	50–59	3	5
	40–49	5	8
	30–39	3	3
	20–29	14	25
	10–19	9	16
	1–9	5	8
Black	90–99	1	2
	70–79	2	3
	60–69	3	5
	50–59	9	16
	40–49	11	19
	30–39	9	16
	20–29	8	14
	10–19	2	3
	1–9	6	10
	0	1	2

TABLE B.2. *(continued)*

	Percent of respondents' patient population	*Number of respondents*	*Percent of respondents*
Hispanic	70–79	1	2
	50–59	4	7
	40–49	15	26
	30–39	10	17
	20–29	12	21
	10–19	4	7
	1–9	7	12
Other	10–19	2	3
	1–9	4	7
	0	46	82
	(no response)	4	7
Risk factors			
Homosexual	90–99	7	12
	80–89	3	5
	70–79	3	5
	60–69	1	2
	50–59	4	7
	40–49	8	14
	30–39	5	8
	20–29	5	8
	10–19	4	7
	1–9	2	3
	0	5	8
Drug user	100	1	2
	90–99	4	7
	80–89	1	2
	70–79	6	10
	60–69	6	10
	50–59	5	8
	40–49	3	5
	30–39	4	7
	20–29	4	7
	10–19	5	8
	1–9	7	12
	0	1	2
Other			
Partner of drug user; blood transfusion recipient	90–99	1	2
	60–69	1	2
	40–49	1	2
	30–39	3	5
	20–29	1	2
	10–19	6	10
	1–9	6	10
	0	28	50
	(no response)	9	16

Appendix C: Comparison of Interview and Survey Responses

Question #1: What prompted you to become involved in HIV care?		
Response	*Number*	*Percent*
1. *Desire to help*		
interview	36	72
survey	39	69
2. *Desire to use skill/talents*		
interview	28	56
survey	33	58
3. *Intrigued with disease*		
interview	24	48
survey	29	51
4. *Personal contact with disease*		
interview	13	26
survey	13	23
5. *Attractive job*		
interview	14	28
survey	11	19
6. *AIDS unit opened*		
interview	4	8
survey	10	10
7. *Commitment to community*		
interview	3	6
survey	3	5
8. *Wanted change*		
interview	6	12
survey	3	5

Question #2: What are the challenges of what you do?

Response	*Number*	*Percent*
1. Patients' emotional needs		
interview	41	82
survey	48	85
2. Comforting patients and families		
interview	26	52
survey	39	60
3. Coping with patient deterioration: physical		
interview	27	54
survey	32	57
4. Coping with patient deterioration: mental		
interview	28	56
survey	33	58
5. Coping with patients' clinical instability		
interview	27	54
survey	32	57
6. Working with colleagues who do not share your philosophy of care		
interview	34	68
survey	32	57
7. Coping with death		
interview	23	46
survey	32	57
8. Sustaining patients' hope		
interview	25	50
survey	31	55
9. Overcoming bureaucratic obstacles		
interview	27	54
survey	31	55
10. Social stigma of disease		
interview	23	46
survey	26	46
11. Maintaining your own emotional balance		
interview	32	64
survey	24	42
12. Working within limitations of care		
interview	27	54
survey	20	35

Question #2: What are the challenges of what you do? (continued)

Response	*Number*	*Percent*
13. Persevering through difficulties and failure		
interview	22	44
survey	16	28
14. Coping with contagion		
interview	4	8
survey	8	14

Question #3: What are the satisfactions of what you do?

Response	*Number*	*Percent*
1. Teaching and counseling		
interview	26	52
survey	43	76
2. Involvement in important work		
interview	34	68
survey	42	75
3. Establishing a personal connection with patients		
interview	36	72
survey	41	73
4. Being able to use every kind of nursing skill		
interview	35	70
survey	36	64
5. Meeting the challenge of clinical care		
interview	30	60
survey	32	57
6. Working with like-minded colleagues		
interview	10	20
survey	27	48

Question #4: Do you meet any ethical issues in your work?

Response	*Number*	*Percent*
1. Access to treatment/drugs		
interview	33	66
survey	35	63
2. DNR's (Do Not Resuscitate orders)		
interview	29	58
survey	30	53
3. Termination of treatment		
interview	32	64
survey	29	51
4. Recognizing the limits of high-tech medical care		
interview	17	34
survey	29	51
5. Maintaining confidentiality		
interview	19	38
survey	28	50
6. Toxic medication		
interview	15	30
survey	25	44
7. Notifying partners/family members		
interview	13	26
survey	20	35
8. Encountering suicide requests		
interview	9	18
survey	19	32
9. Pregnancy decisions by HIV+ patients		
interview	5	10
survey	15	26

Question #5: What keeps you going?

Response	*Number*	*Percent*
1. Pleasure from patient contact		
interview	26	52
survey	45	80
2. Feeling that work is meaningful/needed		
interview	38	76
survey	44	78
3. Personal growth		
interview	37	74
survey	36	64
4. "Making a difference"		
interview	39	78
survey	36	64
5. Commitment to providing health care for all		
interview	33	66
survey	36	64
6. Helping others		
interview	34	68
survey	30	53
7. Clinical interest		
interview	16	32
survey	30	53
8. Having interests outside work		
interview	9	18
survey	23	40
9. Feeling of identification		
interview	7	14
survey	11	19
10. Support from family and friends		
interview	8	16
survey	11	19

Question #10: When you think of being a nurse, does a particular image come to mind, such as:

Response	*Number*	*Percent*
1. *Listening as a patient talks*		
interview	35	70
survey	42	74
2. *Talking with a patient*		
interview	34	68
survey	39	69
3. *Giving physical care*		
interview	30	60
survey	31	55
4. *Sitting by a patient's bed, holding his/her hand*		
interview	26	52
survey	27	48
5. *Walking arm and arm with the patient*		
interview	2	4
survey	20	35
6. *Dispensing medications*		
interview	10	20
survey	20	35
7. *"Being there" for patients*		
interview	4	8
survey	11	19

References

Agan, R. D. 1987. "Intuitive Knowing as a Dimension of Nursing." *Advanced Nursing Science* 10 (1): 63–70.

AIDS ALERT. 1992. "CDC's Expanded AIDS Case Definition Sparks Controversy." *American Health Consultants Publication* 7 (5): 65–71.

Allan, J. D., and B. A. Hall. 1988. "Challenging the Focus on Technology: A Critique of the Medical Model in a Changing Health Care System." *Advanced Nursing Science* 10(3): 22–34.

Anderson, B. 1983. *Imagined Communities*. London: Verso.

Armstrong, D. 1983. "Viral Infections." In *The AIDS Epidemic*, ed. K. Cahill. New York: St. Martin's.

Baer, E. 1991. "Further Thoughts on 'The Feminist Disdain for Nursing.'" Paper delivered October 30, 1991, University of Virginia Health Sciences Center.

Barrett, Elizabeth A. M. 1990. "Introduction." *Visions of Rogers' Science-Based Nursing*. Publication No. 15–2285. New York: National League for Nursing.

Bartlett, L. 1990. "Financing Health Care for Persons with AIDS: Balancing Public and Private Responsibilities." In *AIDS and the Health Care System*, ed. L. Gostin. New Haven, CT: Yale University Press.

Bayer, R. 1990. "Perinatal Transmission of HIV Infection: The Ethics of Prevention." In *AIDS and the Health Care System*, ed. L. Gostin. New Haven, CT: Yale University Press.

Belenky, M. F., B. M. Clinchey, N. R. Goldberger, and J. M. Tarule. 1986. *Women's Ways of Knowing: Development of Self, Voice and Mind*. New York: Basic Books.

Benner, P. 1984. *From Novice to Expert: Excellence and Power in Clinical Nursing*. Menlo Park, CA: Addison-Wesley.

———. 1989. *The Primacy of Caring*. Menlo Park, CA: Addison-Wesley.

Benoit, H. 1955. *The Supreme Doctrine: Psychological Studies in Zen Thought*. New York: Pantheon.

Berger, P. 1990a [1969]. *A Rumor of Angels: Modern Society and the Discovery of the Supernatural*. New York: Doubleday.

———. 1990b [1967]. *The Sacred Canopy*. New York: Doubleday.

Berger, P., B. Berger, and Hansfried Kellner. 1974. *The Homeless Mind*. New York: Random House.

Bruner, J. 1962. *On Knowing: Essays for the Left Hand*. Cambridge, MA: Harvard University Press.

Camus, A. 1948. *The Plague.* Translated by Gilbert Stuart. New York: A. A. Knopf.
Cantwell, A. 1983. *AIDS: The Mystery and the Solution.* Los Angeles: Aries Rising Press.
Cassell, J. 1991. *Expected Miracles: Surgeons at Work.* Philadelphia: Temple University Press.
Centers for Disease Control. *Morbidity and Mortality Weekly Reports,* June 5, 1981. Supplement, September 4, 1987.
Chang, S. 1992. "The New AIDS Case Definition: Implications for San Francisco." *Journal of the American Medical Association* 267: 973–75.
Corea, G. 1992. *The Invisible Epidemic: The Story of Women and AIDS.* New York: HarperCollins.
Crapanzano, V. 1985. *Waiting: The Whites of South Africa.* New York: Random House.
Dumpson, J. R., et al. 1989. "AIDS and Minorities: Strategies for Prevention." International Conference on AIDS. January 4–9. 5: 818 (abstract no. ME023)
Eliade, M. 1954. *The Myth of the Eternal Return.* New York: Pantheon.
Fernandez, J. 1982. "The Dark at the Bottom of the Stairs." In *On Symbols in Anthropology: Essays in Honor of Harry Horjer,* ed. J. Maquet, M. Singer, and M. Spiro. Malibu, CA: Publication of the UCLA Department of Anthropology.
Fiedler, L. 1988. "Images of the Nurse in Fiction and Popular Culture." In *Images of Nurses,* ed. A. H. Jones. Philadelphia: University of Pennsylvania Press.
Foege, W., 1983. "The National Pattern of AIDS." In *The AIDS Epidemic,* ed. K. Cahill. New York: St. Martin's.
Fox, D. M., and E. H. Thomas. 1990. "The Cost of AIDS: Exaggeration, Entitlement, and Economics." In *AIDS and the Health Care System,* ed. L. Gostin. New Haven, CT: Yale University Press.
Fox, R. C., L. H. Aiken, and C. M. Messikomer. 1990. "The Culture of Caring: AIDS and the Nursing Profession." *Milbank Quarterly* 68 (Supplement 2): 226–56.
Freedberg, D. 1989. *The Power of Images: Studies in the History and Theory of Response to Images.* Chicago: University of Chicago Press.
Furth, H. 1987. *Knowledge as Desire: An Essay on Freud and Piaget.* New York: Columbia University Press.
Gadow, S. 1980. "'Existential Advocacy: Philosophical Foundation of Nursing." In *Nursing Images and Ideals,* ed. S. F. Spicker. New York: Springer Publishing.
Gee, G. 1989. "Nurse Attitudes and AIDS." In *Public and Professional Attitudes towards AIDS Patients,* ed. D. E. Rogers and E. Ginzberg. Boulder, CO: Westview Press.
Geertz, C. 1983. *Local Knowledge: Further Essays in Interpretive Anthropology.* New York: Basic Books.
Girardot, N., and M. L. Ricketts. 1982. *Imagination and Meaning: The Scholarly and Literary Worlds of Mircea Eliade.* New York: Seabury Press.
Gorman, E. M. 1986. "The AIDS Epidemic in San Francisco: Epidemiological and Anthropological Perspectives." In *Anthropology and Epidemiology,* ed. C. R. James. Dordrecht, Holland: D. Reidel Publishers.

Harawi, S. J., and C. J. O'Hara. 1989. *Pathology and Pathophysiology of AIDS and HIV-Related Diseases.* London: Chapman and Hall.

Havens, L. 1986. *Making Contact: Uses of Language in Psychotherapy.* Cambridge: Harvard University Press.

Heimhoff, S., and J. Sommer. 1991. "Is the HIV Theory All Wrong?" *CalReport* 8(1): 16–18.

Henderson, V., and B. Harmer. 1939. *Textbook of the Principles and Practice of Nursing.* New York: Macmillan.

Henderson, V. 1990. "Nursing in America: A History of Social Reform." New York: NLN Video.

Jackson, M. 1988. "In the Thrown World: Destiny and Decision in the Thought of Traditional Africa." In *Choice and Morality in Anthropological Perspective.* Albany: SUNY Press.

Jagger, A. 1989. "Love and Knowledge: Emotion in Feminist Epistemology." In *Gender/Body/Knowledge,* ed. A. Jagger. New Brunswick, NJ: Rutgers University Press.

James, W. [1902] 1985. *Varieties of Religious Experience.* Cambridge: Harvard University Press.

Jonsen, A. R. 1990. "The Duty to Treat Patients with AIDS and HIV Infection." In *AIDS and the Health Care System,* ed. L. Gostin. New Haven, CT: Yale University Press.

Journal of the American Medical Association. 1987 258: 9 Supplement 1S.

Journal of the Association of Nurses in AIDS Care 2, no. 4 (1991): 44.

Katz, R. 1963. *Empathy: Its Nature and Uses.* London: MacMillan.

Keller, E. F. 1985. *Reflections on Gender and Science.* New Haven, CT: Yale University Press.

Killip, T. 1989. "Hospitals in NYC: A System under Stress." In *Public and Professional Attitudes Towards AIDS Patients,* ed. D. E. Rogers and E. Ginzberg. Boulder, CO: Westview Press.

Levine, C. 1990. "In and Out of the Hospital." In *AIDS and the Health Care System,* ed. L. Gostin. New Haven, CT: Yale University Press.

Lifton, R. J. 1979. *The Broken Connection: On Death and the Continuity of Life.* New York: Simon and Schuster.

———. 1976. *The Life of the Self.* New York: Simon and Schuster.

Lipson, J. 1991. "A Contemporary Dialogue." In *Qualitative Nursing Research,* ed. J. Morse. Newbury Park, CA: Sage.

Louria, D. B. 1983. "Bacterial and Mycotic Infections." In *The AIDS Epidemic,* ed. K. Cahill. New York: St. Martin's Press.

Ludmerer, K. M. 1989. "Patients Beyond the Pale." In *Public and Professional Attitudes towards AIDS,* ed. D. E. Rogers and E. Ginzberg. Boulder, CO: Westview Press.

Maquet, J. 1986. *The Aesthetic Experience: An Anthropologist Looks at the Visual Arts.* New Haven, CT: Yale University Press.

Malson, L. 1972. *Wolf Children and the Problem of Human Nature.* New York: Monthly Review Press.

Melosh, B. 1982. *The Physician's Hand: Nurses and Nursing in the 20th Century.* Philadelphia, PA: Temple University Press.

Merleau-Ponty, M. 1969. *Eye and Mind: The Essential Writings of Merleau-Ponty,* ed. A. L. Fisher. New York: Harcourt, Brace.

Murray, T. H., and G. M. Aumann. 1987. "Ethical Issues in AIDS." In *AIDS:*

Facts and Issues, ed. V. Gong and N. Rudnick. New Brunswick, NJ: Rutgers University Press.

NYC AIDS Surveillance Report. June 1990. NYC Department of Health Bureau of HIV Program Services: Monthly packet for community based and city-wide organizations.

NYC AIDS Surveillance Update. Fourth Quarter, 1992. NYC Department of Health Office of AIDS Surveillance. Issued January 1993.

Novick, L. F., et al. 1991. "Newborn Seroprevalence Study: Methods and Results." *American Journal of Public Health* 81 (May 1991, Supplement): 15–21.

Paterson, J. G., and L. T. Zderad. 1988. *Humanistic Nursing.* Publication 41–2218 New York: National League for Nursing.

Patton, M. Q. 1990. *Qualitative Evaluation and Research Methods.* Newbury Park, CA: Sage.

Payer, L. 1988. *Medicine and Culture: Varieties of Treatment in the US, England, West Germany, and France.* New York: Henry Holt.

Perin, C. 1988. *Belonging in America.* Madison, WI: University of Wisconsin Press.

Polanyi, M. 1962. *Personal Knowledge.* Chicago: University of Chicago Press.

Reik, T. 1948. *Listening with the Third Ear.* New York: Farrar, Straus.

Reverby, S. 1987. *Ordered to Care.* Cambridge: Cambridge University Press.

Sanday, P. R. 1983. "The Ethnographic Paradigm(s)." In *Qualitative Methodology,* ed. J. Van Maanen. Newbury Park, CA: Sage.

Sarter, B. 1987. "Evolutionary Idealism: A Philosophical Foundation for Holistic Nursing Theory." *Advanced Nursing Science* 9(2): 1–9.

Schwarz, M. R. 1989. "Physicians' Attitudes toward AIDS." In *Public and Professional Attitudes toward AIDS Patients,* ed. D. E. Rogers and E. Ginzberg. Boulder, CO: Westview Press.

Scitovsky, A. 1986. "Medical Care Costs of Patients with AIDS in San Francisco." *Journal of the American Medical Association* 256: 3103–6.

Sloand, E., et al. 1991. "HIV Testing: State of the Art." *Journal of American Medical Association* 266: 2861–66.

Smith, J. 1990. *Patenting the Sun: Polio and the Salk Vaccine.* New York: William Morrow.

Spiegelberg, H. 1976. *The Phenomenological Movement.* The Hague, Netherlands: Martinus Nyhoff.

Starr, P. 1982. *The Social Transformation of American Medicine.* New York: Basic Books.

Surich, Dr. Ilona. 1993. Personal communication, April 19.

Thomas, P. A. "The NYC Perinatal HIV Transmission Study by the NYC Department of Health." International Conference on AIDS, Montreal, Canada. June 8, 1989. Abstract Th.A.O.7.

Tronto, J. C. 1990. "Woman and Caring: What can Feminists Learn about Morality from Caring?" In *Gender/Body/Knowledge,* ed. A. Jagger. New Brunswick, NJ: Rutgers University Press.

Van Maanen, J. 1983. "Reclaiming Qualitative Methods for Institutional Research: A Preface." In *Qualitative Methodology.* Newbury Park, CA: Sage.

Vladeck, B. C. 1989. "The Economics of a Caring Approach." In *Public and Professional Attitudes toward AIDS Patients,* ed. D. E. Rogers and E. Ginzberg. Boulder, CO: Westview Press.

Watson, J. 1988. *Nursing: Human Science and Human Care: A Theory of Nursing.* New York: National League for Nursing.

Watts, F., and M. Williams. 1988. *The Psychology of Religious Knowing*. Cambridge: Cambridge University Press.

Weil, S. 1973 [1951] *Waiting for God*. New York: Harper & Row.

Wolf, Z. R. 1988. *Nurses' Work, The Sacred and The Profane*. Philadelphia, PA: University of Pennsylvania Press.

Index

University of Pennsylvania Press
Studies in Health, Illness, and Caregiving
Joan E. Lynaugh, General Editor

Barbara Bates. *Bargaining for Life: A Social History of Tuberculosis, 1876–1938.* 1992

Michael D. Calabria and Janet Macrae, editors. Suggestions for Thought *by Florence Nightingale: Selections and Commentaries.* 1993

Janet Golden and Charles Rosenberg. *Pictures of Health: A Photographic History of Health Care in Philadelphia.* 1991

Anne Hudson Jones. *Images of Nurses: Perspectives from History, Art, and Literature.* 1987

June S. Lowenberg. *Caring and Responsibility: The Crossroads Between Holistic Practice and Traditional Medicine.* 1989

Peggy McGarrahan. *Transcending AIDS: Nurses and HIV Patients in New York City.* 1994

Elizabeth Norman. *Women at War: The Story of Fifty Military Nurses Who Served in Vietnam.* 1990

Anne Opie. *There's Nobody There: Community Care of Confused Older People.* 1992

Elizabeth Brown Pryor. *Clara Barton, Professional Angel.* 1987

Margarete Sandelowski. *With Child in Mind: Studies of the Personal Encounter with Infertility.* 1993

Zane Robinson Wolf. *Nurses' Work, The Sacred and The Profane.* 1988

This book was set in Baskerville and Eras typefaces. Baskerville was designed by John Baskerville at his private press in Birmingham, England, in the eighteenth century. The first typeface to depart from oldstyle typeface design, Baskerville has more variation between thick and thin strokes. In an effort to insure that the thick and thin strokes of his typeface reproduced well on paper, John Baskerville developed the first wove paper, the surface of which was much smoother than the laid paper of the time. The development of wove paper was partly responsible for the introduction of typefaces classified as modern, which have even more contrast between thick and thin strokes.

Eras was designed in 1969 by Studio Hollenstein in Paris for the Wagner Typefoundry. A contemporary script-like version of a sans-serif typeface, the letters of Eras have a monotone stroke and are slightly inclined.

Printed on acid-free paper.